Toward Fitness

Toward Fitness

Guided Exercise for Those with Health Problems

Robert C. Cantu, M.D., F.A.C.S.

Emerson Hospital,
Concord, Mass.

HUMAN SCIENCES PRESS

72 Fifth Avenue   3 Henrietta Street
NEW YORK, NY 10011 ● LONDON, WC2E 8LU

Printed in the United States of America
0 987654321

Library of Congress Cataloging in Publication Data

Cantu, Robert C
  Toward fitness.

  Bibliography: p. 235
  Includes index.
  1. Exercise. 2. Physical fitness. 3. Exercise therapy. I. Title.
  RA781.C3   613.7'1   LC 79-27686
ISBN 0-87705-496-7

Contents

5

Foreword

It is evident to even the most casual observer that we are in the midst of a "fitness boom" in this country. American men, women, and children of all ages, size, and shapes are turning to activities as diverse as jogging, racquetball, and roller skating for exercise and recreation. Increased leisure time, changed attitudes towards youth, aging, and the social roles of men and women have provided the foundations for this movement. Increased emphasis on exercise in weight loss programs, suggested relationships between regular exercise and longevity, productivity or even improved psychic states have provided further stimulus to many a new jogger or athlete.

Whatever the motivation, these new or renewed athletes and fitness enthusiasts are presenting physicians with a whole new set of problems and questions. In the more traditional sports medicine setting, the injured athlete presented himself to the team doctor, often at the direction of, or at least with the approval of, the coach. If the team was fortunate enough to have an athletic trainer, the athlete may have had an initial assessment by the trainer before seeing the "Doc." The team doctor's primary role was to confirm the diagnosis, estimate the severity of the injury, and, most importantly, prognosticate return to action, in conjunction with an appropriate treatment and rehabilitation program. In the design of a particular rehabilitation program for an athlete in a particular sport, the team doctor could usually count heavily on the resources of coach and trainer for supervision and progression.

Not so with the recreational athlete. Lacking coach, trainer, and often knowledge of either fundamentals of fitness training or even, playing skills in his new sport, his most accessible resource is often the physician dealing with his "sports" injury. While at first exposure questions about running shoes, running surface, type of tennis racquet or ski binding, or even recommended types of hockey helmets or face masks may be both baffling and seem inappropriate questions for a doctor, studies of a number of sports and their injuries confirm the importance of such factors in the occurrence and severity of sports injuries.

A number of books and publications now deal with the problem of the recreational athlete, and the plethora of running books are a reflection of the attention he or she is now receiving. Despite this, it becomes evident that many individuals, not readily included in the categories of school athlete or even recreational athlete, also stand to benefit, often dramatically, from athletic participation.

Dr. Cantu has emphatically and clearly demonstrated the benefits of sports participation for the aged, the diabetic and others who are limited by one or another "handicap," and he has given clear guidelines for progressive and safe conditioning and training for these athletes.

Chapters on sports for the diabetic and the physically handicapped are unique in the field of sports medicine. They represent the most current and comprehensive review of this information now available to the coach, trainer and physician who deals with athletes and their problems.

This carefully researched book can serve as a reference source for sports specialists on these important topics, and at the same time be used by any athlete who wishes to learn about these subjects or deal with some of these problems while engaged in sports training or competition.

We congratulate a fellow physician on a difficult task admirably performed.

Lyle J. Micheli, M.D.
Director, Division of Sports Medicine
Children's Hospital Medical Center
Boston, MA
October 2, 1979

Introduction

As the most sports-minded and exercise-conscious people in the history of Western civilization since the ancient Greeks and Romans, we take good health and physical fitness for granted. For many Americans, sports and exercise are a way of life. We are members of softball teams, we bowl regularly, we belong to tennis clubs, and now we have become interested in jogging and long distance running. Yet perhaps only a minority of Americans—at least adult Americans—should engage in physical activities without giving a second thought to their bodies. These are the nation's "healthy elite," people who have been exercising routinely since childhood.

To date, it has been to this "healthy elite" that nearly all advice on physical conditioning and sports participation has been directed. For example, nearly every book on the subject assumes that the reader is healthy. The only concession this literature makes to those people with health problems is the standard one-sentence statement that they should have a physical examination before following an exercise program.

Yet most Americans, while they love sports and would like to be more physically active, do not have completely healthy bodies and must proceed with caution. I call these people—and I include myself in this group—"physically disadvantaged." *We are not disabled* in the sense of being totally incapacitated, but we do have health problems that require regular care and supervision and that must be considered in any exercise or sports program we undertake. In many instances we have multiple health problems, say, heart disease, hypertension, obesity, and diabetes—each of which must be considered separately and in combination when playing sports or exercising.

It is for myself and other "physically disadvantaged" Americans—*and we are the vast majority in today's adult* population—that this book was researched and written. The basic assumption underlying every line in it is that the "physically disadvantaged" can and should achieve physical fitness—indeed that our lives can be every much as active and fun-filled as the "healthy elite."

In the chapters that follow, an exercise and sports program has been designed to meet each of the major health problems that restrict the lives of Americans today. It is important to emphasize again that few of us have just one physical disadvantage. Usually, we must cope with several problems—which is especially true of the elderly population. Therefore, keep all of your health problems in mind as you read this book and evolve an exercise program that meets your particular needs.

Who are America's "physically disadvantaged"? They include the following: diabetics (10 percent of today's population); coronary patients (including survivors of the single greatest killer in the modern world, heart attacks, and those suffering from hypertension and atherosclerosis); and stroke victims.

Other Americans who are likely to be physically disadvantaged are those with persistent back ailments, as well as those who are overweight, elderly, or simply sedentary. Ruptured or herniated discs, spondylolisthesis (a slippage of the vertebra out of perfect alignment), and the far more common chronic back strain, are injuries that intrude dramatically into our lives, restricting mobility and preventing physical exercise. A bad back can bring almost unmanageable levels of pain and cause severe depression.

The obese are another group of physically—and often emotionally—disabled Americans. Excess weight is frequently an indirect cause of death and it usually discourages physical fitness. The aged must also be categorized as physically disadvantaged. Two-thirds of all health care dollars are spent on those over 45 years of age. This population, which is almost entirely sedentary and neglectful of physical fitness, is increasing rapidly and represents a built-in "time bomb" for medical care spending.

Finally, large numbers of Americans are physically disadvantaged from simple but long-term neglect of their bodies. Years of inactivity will inevitably develop into a health problem. We who let ourselves go for years, without concern, begin at about 40 to lose confidence in our health and physical fitness. Growing fears of sudden health problems prevent us from participating in new activities. We are unsure of our bodies and fearful that sudden exertion may precipitate a coronary or stroke. These people, without pathological symptoms but with fear of using their bodies, must be recognized as physically disadvantaged.

The physical disadvantages discussed in this book are determined both by genetics and environment. We are all born with a set of genes that may be thought of as a *"biological clock,"* a fixed period of time on earth inherited from our parents. Because we did not pick our parents, our genetic makeup or "biological clock" is something over which we have no control. It follows that people with excellent inherited protection can neglect their bodies and live longer than others who neglect their bodies but have weaker genetic protection. Most of us, however, cheat ourselves out of months, years, or even decades of good health by inappropriate life habits.

It is shocking to realize that more than seven hundred thousand Americans die annually of heart attacks. Certainly some of these people had unpreventable illnesses, but the majority were the physically disadvantaged—due in part to their genetic makeup—who raced to their deaths through a lifestyle of self-pollution and inactivity. Tragically, this style not only shortens life but, what is perhaps more important, it deprives us of maximum daily enjoyment and productivity.

In the pages that follow, the physical disadvantages resulting from diabetes, heart attack, stroke, back trouble, obesity, age, and prolonged inactivity will be examined in depth. Individual exercise programs have been tailored to each disadvantage. Since many readers suffer from multiple problems, age, obesity, and coronary problems, for example, readers are advised to examine the entire book in order to be aware of how the diseases are interrelated and to determine which programs best fit their special needs. This also will afford the best opportunity to avoid physical ailments in the future that you do not have now. However, for those of you with a single ailment, the following guide will allow you to use this book most expediently.

Everyone should read the Introduction, Chapter 1, on the Cardiovascular System, Chapter 2 on Nutrition, Chapter 10, and the Appendix.

The *obese* should add Chapter 3 to this list and, once a desired weight is achieved, may progress to either Chapter 8 or 9, depending on your age.

For the *diabetic,* Chapter 4 is to be added to the Introduction and Chapters 1, 2, 10 and the Appendix. In addition, either Chapter 8 or 9 is to be included depending again on whether you are over or under 60 years of age. Age sixty is not a magic figure and, thus, those who are not yet sixty, but are severely physically unfit, may wish to start with Chapter 9 and six or more months later progress to Chapter 8.

Those with a *back problem* should add Chapter 5 to the core chapters (Introduction, 1, 2, 10 and Appendix). Once the back problem is overcome, then progress to Chapter 8 or 9 as discussed for the diabetic.

The *disabled* (upper and lower limb amputee, quadra and paraplegic, blind and deaf) will add Chapter 6 to the core chapters and the *post-heart attack* patient adds Chapter 7. After a suitable time period, about six to eight months, some from either group may safely be able to progress to Chapter 8 or 9.

The *inactive* but *under 60 group* include Chapter 8 with the core chapters and *senior citizens, 60* and above, add Chapter 9.

This is a streamlined plan to allow you to work out an exercise fitness program, rapidly and safely, specifically tailored to your own physical disadvantages. While I encourage you to use the book in this manner initially; since your needs may change in the future, I strongly urge that eventually you read the entire book. It may well avert future physical problems and will certainly give you insight into the common afflictions of our middle and later years.

Every man is the builder of a temple, called his body. . . . We are all sculptors and painters, and our material is our own flesh and blood and bones.

Henry David Thoreau

1

The Tree Trunk of Life: A Healthy Cardiovascular System

Endurance exercise is to the body what reading and writing are to the mind.

R. C. Cantu

$\mathcal{F}$or those of us who suffer from the physical disadvantages of diabetes, heart disease, back problems, obesity, age, or prolonged inactivity, the road back to a vigorous life begins with a fit cardiovascular system. For all people, the cardiovascular system is the *tree trunk of life*. It consists of the heart, arteries, and veins and it conducts our blood, containing life-essential oxygen and nutrients, to all of our body cells.

Physically disadvantaged individuals usually suffer from some impairment of their cardiovascular system. Frequently, the disruption is sudden and severe, perhaps a major blockage of a coronary artery (heart attack) or a cerebral artery occlusion or rupture (stroke). Others more fortunate may be aware of a deteriorating system only by the tell-tale signs of excessive fatigue, shortness of breath, or chest pain following physical activity. Heart attacks not only kill and disable more people in the Western world than any other affliction, but as affluent life spreads to the non-Western world, the incidence of heart attack climbs there, also.

GENETICS AND HEALTH PROBLEMS

The root cause of cardiovascular impairment may be attributed to our genes as indicated by prior family history.* Knowing about our family's health past will explain much about our own constitutions. Indeed, our own life expectancy (before calculating the negative factors of bodily abuse and self-pollution or the positive factors of exercise and proper nutrition) can be inferred from the longevity of close relatives. If anyone in our immedi-ate family—great-grandparents, grandparents, parents, aunts, uncles—died at an early age of a coronary or stroke, that should serve as a warning to us. Physically disadvantaged persons with this kind of family past should begin an exercise program immediately in order to resist the genetic weaknesses they have inherited.

Beside stroke and heart disease, diabetes is also an inherited illness that contributes to cardiovascular disorders. Diabetes is characterized by a deficiency of the insulin-secreting cells of the pancreas. The major complications of this disease involve an acceleration of the process of arteriosclerosis of our vascular system. The diabetic is at increased risk for stroke, heart attack, renal and retinal vascular disease.

*Cardiovascular impairment can also be non-genetically related. For example, prolonged inactivity will eventually erode cardiovascular efficiency.

Three basic factors are involved in optimal diabetic control: diet, medicatiòn, and exercise. Only recently has the medical profession acknowledged the importance of sustained, daily cardiovascular exercise in the management of diabetes. Following intelligent, appropriate physical conditioning, no exercise program or specific sport need be denied the diabetic. Indeed, virtually all our major sports have diabetic superstars such as Bill Tilden and Ham Richardson of tennis, Jim "Catfish Hunter" of baseball, and Bobby Clarke of hockey. Chapter 4 in this book is devoted to diabetics and their exercise needs.

Thus far we have discussed family history and diabetes as risk factors for coronary disease. The Framingham Study started in 1968 and sponsored by the United States Public Health Service closely followed 5,000 residents (2,-336 males and 2,873 females) of a Massachusetts town to study coronary disease (9–13). Men with elevated cholesterol levels, who had hypertension or diabetes, and smoked, had 10 times more coronary artery disease than the national average. If all those factors were absent, the likelihood was reduced to one-third the standard risk. Thus, very clearly, a man with elevation of blood cholesterol, hypertension, and diabetes, has a greatly increased chance of a heart attack. After menopause, women have an equal risk for heart attacks as men.

Cigarette smoking has been shown to significantly increase the risk of coronary disease. The incidence of sudden death is nearly 400 percent greater in cigarette smokers. In the experience of the Toronto Rehabilitation Centre, under Medical Director Dr. Terrence Kavanaugh, the incidence of recurrent fatal heart attack in smokers was 1.3 percent.(14) This center uses endurance training through a progressive walking-jogging program for its post heart attack patients, several of whom have progressed to running marathons. Dr. Kavanaugh states that most of the deaths were in patients who, despite admonitions, had not stopped smoking cigarettes. (Pipe and cigar smokers resemble non-smokers in heart attack incidence, as long as they are not ex-cigarette smokers.)

Obesity has also been shown to be a risk factor for heart attacks. It rarely occurs, however, except in association with one or more of the other risk factors such as diabetes, hypertension, high blood cholesterol, or inactivity. Thus, obesity appears to be a risk factor mainly because of the other conditions it predisposes you to.

Emotional stress and a personality characterized by cardiologists Friedman and Rosenman as competitive, excessively ambitious, impatient with delay, compulsive, and never satisfied with attaining any achievement have been implicated as possible risk factors for coronary disease.(7) The findings are far from conclusive as multiple studies in the United States and abroad indicate no correlation between responsibility at work and coronary disease. But the personality described is also frequently associated with other risk factors, such as smoking.

Inactivity is the final risk factor for heart attack. Professor Jeremy Morris of the British Research Council, first drew attention to this fact in 1953 with his report in *The Lancet* entitled "Coronary Heart Disease and Physical Activity of Work."(16) He studied the incidence of heart disease in the London Transport Department workers and found that bus conductors, who averaged twenty-four trips per hour up and down the winding staircase of the moving double decker bus, had one-third less heart disease than the sedentary bus drivers.

In 1973, Morris again reported in *The Lancet* the beneficial effects of leisure-time exercise in 17,000 British civil servants.(17) Morris concluded, "habitual vigorous exercise during leisure time reduces the incidence of coronary heart disease in middle age among sedentary male workers. Vigorous activities which are normal for such men are sufficient. Training of the heart and cardiovascular system is one of the mechanisms of protection against common risk factors and the disease."

More recently, in 1977, Dr. Ralph S. Paffenbarger, Jr., has reported that the risk of heart attack is significantly reduced in men engaging in strenuous sports, while "casual" sports seemed to have no beneficial effect. His research involved 17,000 male alumni of Harvard University aged 35–74, who were studied for 6–10 years. Heart attack rates were shown to decline with increasing activity. This trend held true for all ages and for both non-fatal and fatal attacks. The more calories the men spent in total activity in a week, the less risk of heart attack. It appeared that 2,000 calories expended per week in exercise was required to protect against heart attack. This protective effect from being active seemed to hold regardless of whether the men had other risk factors such as cigarette smoking, hypertension, obesity, or poor heredity with a parental heart attack history. Among the strenuous sports affording protection, Dr. Paffenbarger listed running, swimming, basketball, handball, and squash. "Casual" sports that afforded no protection included golf, bowling, baseball, softball, and volleyball.(18, 19)

In keeping with the benefits of daily physical activity, it is of note to reflect on the three regions of the world most renowned for longevity, the Ecuadorian Andes, the Karakoran mountains in Kashmir, and the Agkazia region of southern Soviet Union. In these three regions ages of 100 or more are not uncommon and heart attacks are quite rare. Researchers have noted that diets vary and that drinking is common among the aged. In all three regions, the people assumed they would live to an old age and work literally until they dropped. The nature of their work involves heavy physical labor and frequent sustained walking over hilly terrain. While working, these people expend 400–800 calories daily. Objective physical examination showed a very high degree of cardiovascular fitness. Therefore, substantial evidence now exists that, cardiovascular fitness from work, or, of necessity, from a formal exercise program, prevents heart attack and increases longevity.

Thus, the major definite risk factors for heart disease among younger men and both sexes after 50, include hypertension, hypercholesterolemia, cigarette smoking, diabetes, heredity, obesity, and physical inactivity.

WHO RULES THE BODY?

Niccolo Machiavelli said in *The Prince* that, "Fortune is the arbiter of half the things we do, leaving the other half or so to be controlled by ourselves." While he was concerned with the health of the State, his wisdom also applies to a healthy body. Everyone can benefit from physical fitness. But for those of us who have become disadvantaged through a faulty genetic inheritance, a physical fitness program is *essential* if we are to extract the maximum time from our biological clocks.

We are never too old to begin a program of cardiovascular improvement. At birth, our vascular system—blood vessels—are largely free of fatty deposits, but with each day of life, accumulation of deposits is occurring. Osborn, an English researcher, showed that early signs of disease can be detected in the coronary arteries of children as young as 5 years, and that, between 16 and 20 years over half the population has atherosclerosis of the coronary arteries.(14) Autopsy studies of Korean War casualties show that many soldiers already had very significant arteriosclerosis before the age of 25. This should demonstrate that a total fitness program is desirable from the cradle to the grave. However, it is never too late to begin a program as indicated by the fact that post–heart attack patients have even completed full 26 mile, 385 yard marathons. Furthermore, recent studies have shown a reduction in previous arteriosclerosis with cardiovascular endurance training.(2)

SELECTING A PHYSICAL FITNESS PROGRAM

What is physical fitness? What are the best cardiovascular exercises for you? The answers to these two questions are basic to your fitness program. First, to understand fitness it is necessary to know a bit of the physiology of exercise. (This subject will be dealt with in more detail later in the diabetes chapter.)

Our atmosphere on earth contains 21 percent oxygen. Our bodies require a constant supply of oxygen to survive, and within a few minutes of its deprivation, the cells of our body begin to die, beginning with the most sensitive: the brain.

Oxygen is extracted from the air we breath in our lungs. Our breathing is controlled automatically by a feedback system from our brain. Specific cells in the brain respond to the blood levels of oxygen and when the content falls below a critical level, the brain sends impulses through its nerves to the chest wall, diaphragm, and heart. This causes one to breath more deeply and rapidly. The increased heart rate results in a greater volume of blood being delivered to the lungs to acquire the increased oxygen being supplied.

Our lungs consist of ever-smaller air passages: the major bronchi, smaller bronchioles, and tiny, terminal air sacs known as alveoli. The walls of the alveoli contain fine, hair-like capillary blood vessels which are part of the lungs' circulation. In accordance with the laws of physics, gases pass through a permeable membrane (our capillary blood vessel's walls) from a region of highest concentration to a region of lower concentration. Thus, oxygen passes from the alveoli to the capillary blood vessels. In the capillary blood vessels, most of the oxygen (some remains freely dissolved in the blood) combines with a protein substance in our red blood cells called *hemoglobin.*

In this form, it is carried away from the lungs to the left side of the heart. From there it is pumped through the arterial system. The arteries branch into smaller and smaller vessels until they end in capillaries, this time in muscles and the other tissues of the body. In this way, oxygen-rich blood is delivered to active oxygen-poor muscles. There the oxygen separates from the hemoglobin under the influence of various environmental conditions (including heat of muscle contraction, acidity, and presence of myoglobin). The net result is that the muscle is supplied with oxygen and the de-oxygenated blood returns through the veins to the right side of the heart, from which it is pumped to the lungs to repeat the whole cycle again (see Figure 1-1).

Muscles exert their work by contracting—or shortening—in length with an interlocking action by which their two component protein fibrils—*actin* and *myosin*—slide together. Energy is required to initiate and continue this work. The immediate source of energy to initiate the sliding movement of actin and myosin is a chemical substance known as *adenosine triphosphate* or ATP which releases energy when converted to *adenosine diphosphate* (ADP) (see Figure 1-2). The body must replace its local store of muscle ATP for as long as muscle contraction occurs.

The source of energy for the reconversion of ADP to ATP comes from the food we eat. The major source of short term energy involves the breakdown of *glycogen* to *glucose* which is oxidized or combined with oxygen to form carbon dioxide and water. A plentiful supply of oxygen is required for the oxidation of glucose. In the absence of sufficient oxygen, breakdown of glycogen halts part way, less ATP is synthesized, and a toxic substance known as *lactic acid* is produced. Lactic acid accumulates in the muscles and the bloodstream and produces the sensation of fatigue and muscle soreness. High levels actually block the formation of more ATP and eventually may lead to the cessation of muscle contraction altogether.

The type of exercise which leads to *anaerobic* or oxygen-deficient activity, in which the effort outstrips the

Figure 1–1

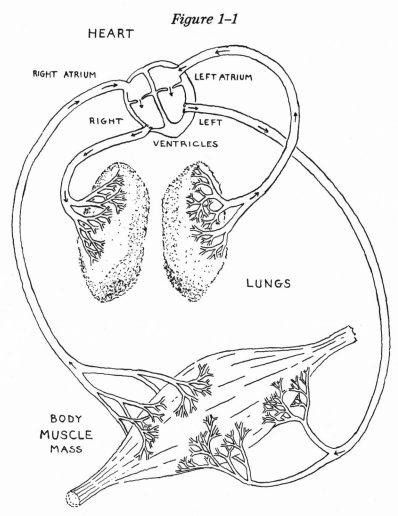

HEART

RIGHT ATRIUM

LEFT ATRIUM

RIGHT

LEFT

VENTRICLES

LUNGS

BODY
MUSCLE
MASS

body's ability to supply oxygen, is characterized by swimming underwater or sprinting. It can be done for only a few minutes. Some individuals do have greater ability to sustain higher levels of anaerobic work than others; however, world champions, whether sprinters, or distance performers, are *born* not made. Training will improve both speed and ability to incur large oxygen debts, but the po-

Figure 1–2

LOHMANN REACTION

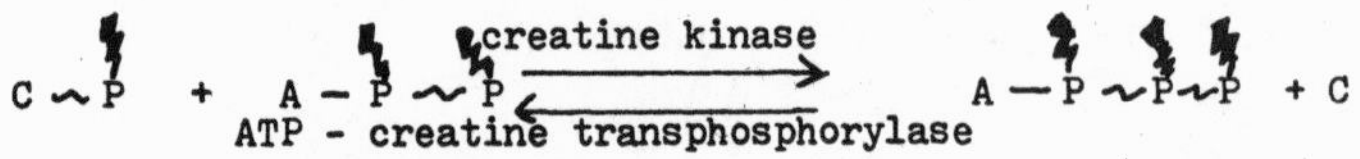

$$C \sim P \ + \ A - P \sim P \ \xrightarrow[\text{ATP - creatine transphosphorylase}]{\text{creatine kinase}} \ A - P \sim P \sim P \ + \ C$$

C P = creatine phosphate

A P P + A D P (adenosine diphosphate)

creatine kinase = enzyme in muscle that allows the reaction
to proceed to the right

A T P - creatine transphosphorylase = enzyme in muscle that
allows reaction to pro-
ceed to the left

A P P P = A T P (adenosine triphosphate)

C = creatine

tential world record holder is born with a greater potential for anaerobic metabolism.

The type of exercise we can sustain is *aerobic*—exercise in which the oxygen supply is sufficient. The more oxygen one can use per minute, the higher is one's ability to perform aerobic-type or endurance-type work. The maximal oxygen we can use per minute is one's *maximal oxygen consumption* (or (VO_2 max) expressed as ml. of oxygen per kilogram of body weight per minute). Fitness is defined in terms of our maximal oxygen consumption.

Included in the oxygen transport system are our lungs, adequate hemoglobin in the blood, an efficient chemical system in our muscles, and the movement of blood by our pump, the heart. Assuming one does not have lung disease and is not anemic, from a practical point of view we can say that one's maximal oxygen consumption is primarily a measure of one's maximal cardiac output. *Thus above all, in answer to the first question, physical fitness is de-*

termined by the efficiency of the heart and is measured by our ability to consume oxygen.

Now let us address ourselves to the second question: what are the best cardiovascular exercises for you? It has been said that the best exercise is the one you most enjoy, as it is the one you will most likely continue to pursue. Characteristics in some exercises are most desirable and make them more efficient than others.

The primary objective is *sustained vigorous exercise pursued for a length of time sufficient to burn an excess of 400 calories.* The activity should increase your heart rate to approximately 75–80 percent of its maximal potential in order to bring about cardiovascular improvement. For most of us this means a pulse rate of around 120–150 per minute to achieve the increased endurance. This is also, practically speaking, a 75–80 percent maximal oxygen consumption. To exceed 80 percent of maximal cardiac output as measured by pulse rate, may lead to inadequate oxygenation, ie., anaerobic metabolism and tissue damage, and thus should be avoided. In reality, most exercise is achieved at lower pulse rates.

Sustained exercise means it must be done continuously, without stopping. If you plan to exercise for 30 minutes or more, do not stop once during that period of time. Sports such as tennis, with the delays between points, or football, with the huddle between every play, rank low as a fitness exercise.

The second desirable characteristic is that the exercise be rhythmical, with the muscles alternately contracting and relaxing. This implies steady, flowing movements that contain no stops or starts once underway. Included in this group are walking, jogging, running, hiking, cross-country skiing, swimming, bicycle riding, and rowing a boat. You can readily see that golf, baseball, football, tennis, etc. with the stop-and-go type activity rate poorly.

The third feature of efficient exercise involves the ability to increase the work load as your level of fitness increases. With increased fitness the same activity that initially caused a pulse rate of 140 may now produce an increase to only 100. Thus the activity must be made progressively more difficult. This can be accomplished in one of two ways. One can slowly *increase the overall rate* at which he or she carrys out the exercise. The progress should be accomplished in many small steps. Or one can *introduce intervals of a faster pace alternating with a slower pace.* The faster pace should be sufficiently vigorous so that you incur an oxygen debt; then switch to a slower pace in order to replenish your oxygen debt. Competitive athletes use interval training extensively, (1, 20) but most of you will probably prefer to increase your pace slowly at a comfortable rate as your fitness progresses.

The last feature of effective exercise is endurance. *Exercise must be sustained for at least half an hour and if possible, up to one hour to produce maximum results.* It also should be done at least four days a week, preferably five. The added advantage of exercising every day is only another percent or two of fitness; except for the diabetic, daily exercise is not necessary, but of course is not discouraged, either.

WHAT ARE THE PHYSIOLOGICAL EFFECTS OF INCREASED CARDIOVASCULAR FITNESS?

The first sign of increased cardiovascular fitness is slowing of the heart rate. This slowing, *bradycardia,* is experienced both at rest and at exercise. That is, with a specific amount of exertion, the fit person's heart rate will increase but will still be far slower than the non-fit person's. The second effect of cardiovascular fitness is that the heart pumps more blood with each contraction. The volume of blood pumped per heart beat, called *stroke volume,* is thus increased. The heart is therefore working more powerfully and efficiently. It can be thought of as loafing along at a slower pace doing the same amount of work, *(cardiac output),* because each contraction is more forceful.

The precise physiological explanation for endurance exercise induced bradycardia remains unknown. The heart rate is the net effect of the impulses of two sets of nerves. The nerves which *speed up* the heart rate are the *sympathetic nerves* and the nerves which *slow* the heart rate are *parasympathetic nerves.* These nerves are part of the autonomic nervous system which operates automatically, without any conscious thought. The digestive tract, various internal glands, as well as the heart and blood vessels are controlled by this division of the nervous system that operates automatically.

At times of fear or anxiety, the sympathetic nervous system takes over and the heart rate increases, causing an increase in blood pressure. Regular endurance exercise resulting in cardiovascular fitness means an increase in parasympathetic activity at rest and a decrease in sympathetic activity with exertion. Thus there is a slowing of the heart rate and lowering of blood pressure both at rest and with exercise. With this parasympathetic predominance the heart is less susceptible to the influence of sudden shocks, stresses, and anxiety provoking situations that confront us daily.

The heart is a muscle and as it increases in strength it enlarges. The young endurance athlete, the long distance runner, swimmer, or cyclist, will experience an enlargement of the heart. I mention this only because in years past many ultra-fit young endurance athletes were labeled as "abnormal" and worse yet, kept from competing because their "hearts were too big." This enlargement is normal: it involves primarily the main pumping chamber of the heart, the left ventricle, and bears no resemblance to the enlargement of a failing heart. The youth should only be encouraged to continue his training. Now that many people in their forties and beyond are rigorously exercising, we may see some cardiac enlargement in this age group as well.

As the heart enlarges in size, a proportional increase

occurs in the diameter and number of branches of the main coronary arteries as well as the tiny capillary blood vessels. These large coronary arteries have the distinct advantage of being so large as to render them extremely unlikely of occlusion—or blockage—by even a lifetime's deposit of fatty atheromatous material. Dr. Thomas Bassler, a pathologist and past President of the American Medical Joggers Association, has stated that he has never seen a documented heart attack from a coronary occlusion in an individual who has gotten his or her endurance fitness to the point of being able to complete a marathon.(3)

The heart receives its own blood flow between contractions. This period is called *diastole;* the period of contraction is termed *systole.* The slower the heart rate the longer the "resting period," diastole. The greater the length of diastole, the greater is the blood flow to the heart muscle. Thus, another advantage of fitness exercise is that the heart gets a greater blood supply. Fitness also produces a reduction in the oxygen requirements of the heart. Therefore, the individual with cardiovascular fitness is living far within his or her cardiac reserve. They are thus afforded a large margin of protection from the daily stresses of life that may challenge a less fit heart.

I have already mentioned that increased cardiovascular fitness is associated with a decrease in blood pressure both at rest and with exertion. Since the deposit of atheromatous material is accelerated by an increase in blood pressure as in stroke and heart attack, increased fitness is obviously a deterrent to each of those conditions. A heart attack can frequently be traced to a specific unaccustomed heavy physical exertion or great anxiety—provoking situation. Each of these situations increases heart rate and thus, blood pressure. If pre-existing disease is present, the workload on the heart may outstrip its ability to supply itself with adequate oxygen during diastole, and the result is a heart attack.

Isometric muscle contractions, such as straining to lift

a heavy object, are especially hazardous since they cause an abrupt and dramatic rise in blood pressure. Fit individuals, however, can carry out heavy physical tasks or be exposed to anxiety—provoking situations with very little increase in heart rate or blood pressure. It has also been shown in a number of different studies(14) that people who regularly engage in heavy physical exercise have less increase in blood pressure with advancing years. Several forms of hypertension have even been attributed to too little physical activity (see Kraus and Raab's book *Hypokinetic Disease.*) (14)

In addition to direct improvements in the heart, endurance fitness brings other benefits. It has been shown that such fitness lengthens clotting time and, in essence, makes the blood less "sticky." This means that occlusion of blood vessels is less likely and that circulation is more efficient because the blood can "slide" through all the vessels with greater ease. Heavy exercise has also been shown to lower the serum blood cholesterol level, which protects against a diet relatively high in saturated fats. Studies in the last two years have shown a reversal of the size of arteriosclerotic plaques when the previously elevated blood pressure and blood cholesterol were reduced to normal levels.(2)

In summary, the beneficial effects of endurance training on the normal, middle-aged heart include a slowing of the heart rate (bradycardia), prolongation of diastole and thus increased blood flow to the heart muscle, increase in stroke volume and thus more efficient and powerful work of the heart muscle, reduced blood pressure, reduced clotting time and viscosity—or stickiness—of the blood, and a decrease in blood fats and their deposition in the body's blood vessels. (See Table 1–1.)

Dr. Kenneth Cooper in his *Aerobics,* subsequently *The New Aerobics,* and most recently *The Aerobics Way,* presents a readily understood method of quantifying exercise. He provides charts which give point values for different types of exercises.(4,5,6) For example, swimming 250 yards in five minutes is worth 2 points, while playing

Table 1-1
Positive Influences of Chronic Endurance Physical Exercise

Blood Vessels and Chemistry
Increase blood oxygen content
Increase blood cell mass and blood volume
Increase fibrinolytic capability
Increase efficiency of peripheral blood distribution and return
Increase blood supply to muscles and more efficient exchange of oxygen
  and carbon dioxide
Reduce serum triglycerides and cholesterol levels
Reduce platelet cohesion or stickiness
Reduce systolic and diastolic blood pressure, especially when elevated
Reduce glucose intolerance

Heart
Increase strength of cardiac contraction (myocardial efficiency)
Increase blood supply (collateral) to heart
Increase size of coronary arteries
Increase size of heart muscle
Increase blood volume (stroke volume) per heart beat
Increase heart rate recovery after exercise
Reduced heart rate at rest
Reduced heart rate with exertion
Reduced vulnerability to cardiac arrythmias

Lungs
Increased blood supply
Increase diffusion of O_2 and CO_2
Increase functional capacity during exercise
Reduce non functional volume of lung

Endocrine (Glandular) and Metabolic Function
Increase tolerance to stress
Increase glucose tolerance
Increase thyroid function
Increase growth hormone production
Increase lean muscle mass
Increase enzymatic function in muscle cells
Increase functional capacity during exercise (muscle oxygen uptake ca-
  pacity)
Reduce body fat content
Reduce chronic catecholamine production
Reduce neurohumeral overreaction

Neural and Psychic
Reduce strain and nervous tension resulting from psychological stress
Reduction in tendency for depression
Euphoria or "joie de vivre" experienced by many

handball for thirty minutes is worth 4½ points. Dr. Cooper contends that, if people accumulate 30–34 points per week they can consider themselves physically fit. Dr. Cooper's ideas as to how total physical fitness is achieved are summarized in two basic principles: first, if one exercises 12–20 minutes per day, it must be exercise vigorous enough to sustain a heart beat of 150 per minute; second, if the exercise fails to reach that level, it must be sustained for a longer period of time to be equally beneficial.

In concluding this chapter, it is important to state again that cardiovascular fitness is realized only by a sustained steady increase in heart rate for periods of at least 30 minutes, four times a week. Ideally the activity should be rhythmic and the intensity increased as fitness improves.

With the objective of exercise as sustained increase in heart rate, it is apparent that any activity done at an accelerated rate can be used, from running to vacuuming the floor. However, not all sports meet this criterion. Tennis, for example, rates quite poorly as physical exercise because of the frequent standing around between points. Likewise golf, walking, baseball, football, weight lifting, and even calisthenics do not achieve a sustained increase in heart rate unless maintained for regular periods with short rest intervals. Other sports activities such as downhill skiing, squash, handball, racquetball, and basketball generate a moderate level of cardiovascular exercise but the activity is not continuous. The activities that achieve maximal cardiovascular exercise levels include running, stationary running, cross-country skiing, swimming, rowing, and cycling.

The *amount* of exercise required for good cardiovascular fitness varies with the exercise pursued. From the maximal group (see Table 1–2), it can be achieved by exercise periods of 30 minutes duration, four or five times a week. From the moderate group, the same cardiovascular fitness requires sixty minutes. The minimal group may be part of a total fitness program, but will not contribute significantly to cardiovascular fitness. Regardless of the activity, we should push ourselves to the point of breathing deeply, but not gasping for breath. For all readers, whatever your particular physical disadvantage may be, *the primary goal of your exercise program should be a fit cardiovascular system.* The chapters that follow outline exercise programs that provide a way for individuals to overcome their particular physical disadvantages, and to achieve this deserved state of cardiovascular fitness.

Table 1–2

Below is a table that categorizes both in terms of aerobic points and calories expended per hour in the exercises previously discussed.

Type of exercise	Aerobic points/hour	Calories burned/hour	
Cross-country skiing	60	900 (10 mph)	MAXIMAL
Running (10 mph)	60	900	
Swimming (1 mph)	48	600 (0.5 mph)	
Stationary running	24 (80–90 steps per minute)	400	
Boxing	22	650	
Cycling	20 (20 mph)	660 (13 mph)	
Hockey	11	600	MODERATE
Basketball	11	600	
Racquetball	11	600	
Football	6	360	
Downhill skiing	6	350	
Tennis	5 (singles)	420	
Walking	3	210	MINIMAL
Baseball	2	270	
Golf	0.75	250	
Weight lifting	Minimal	300	
Isometrics	0	160	

2

Nutrition and Physical Exercise

... leave gormandizing; know the grave doth gape for thee thrice wider than for other men

William Shakespeare (1564–1616)

*T*here is obviously a close relationship between diet and nutrition and physical exercise. First of all, people who exercise regularly make heavy demands on their body's reserves of fluids and energy. They must be aware of the special dietary and nutritional needs that they create as a result of their exercise program. The ordinary diet must be adjusted and supplemented if we are to realize the maximum benefit from our exercise program.

Furthermore, for people who are overweight and/or suffer from a chronic ailment like diabetes or heart disease, exercise alone will not solve—or greatly relieve—the condition. To achieve a maximum level of physical conditioning in the shortest possible time and a maximal control of their chronic ailment, a carefully regulated diet must be combined with the daily program of exercise.

Let us explore, then, the long range effects of diet—especially the American diet—on our general physical condition. Then we will outline the proper diet for those of us with physical ailments who are following the exercise programs outlined in this book.

DIETARY OBJECTIVES FOR AMERICANS

The recent McGovern Committee that studied American dietary habits concluded that Americans eat too much. And they eat the wrong things. They consume too much meat, saturated fat, cholesterol, sugar, and salt. At the same time, they don't eat enough fruit, grains—especially whole grain products—vegetables, and unsaturated fat. The committee urged that the public be educated nutritionally to increase its consumption of fresh, whole foods and to sharply reduce its intake of fat and sugar.

The suggestions of the committee, although physiologically sound, will not be easily implemented in this country. It's advice that runs counter to longstanding ethnic and cultural eating patterns. Implementation would also cause heavy financial losses to major food producers and manufacturers who control food advertising—especially advertising of sugar-laden cereals that appeal to children. These companies will not welcome an attempt to change the financially successful sugared status quo.

Despite the expected resistance from cultural markets and big business, the recommended dietary changes will ultimately be realized. Today, Americans are more fitness-conscious than ever before, and the enthusiasm is far from cresting. More Americans today are pursuing strenuous physical exercise than ever before. Dietary responsibility is a necessary by-product of such concern for physical well being. The old adage that you are what you eat is poignantly pertinent today.

Losing Weight Through Diet and Exercise

Body weight is lost when one or more of the body's essential substances is decreased, thus reducing total body mass. Short term weight loss can be effected by loss of water, fat, protein, or glycogen. Such weight loss occurs frequently during periods of strenuous exercise, as we will discuss below. Longer term weight loss however, also depletes the supply of minerals in the bone and soft tissues of the body.

Actually, weight loss is a simple biological process that is related to the protein, glycogen and water that exist in the body. Every gram of protein or glycogen has coupled with it approximately 3 to 4 grams of water. When a deficit of protein or glycogen occurs, there follows water loss as well. Presently, it is not established that there is any water loss when triglycerides or free fatty acids are mobilized from adipose cells.

Until recently, diabetologists believed that on the average, one pound (0.45 kg) of body weight loss corresponded to the burning of about 3,500 calories. This figure was derived from a value suggesting that 98 percent of the calories burned were derived from body fat. Studies now show that during the first several weeks of dietary restriction, weight loss is far in excess of the caloric deficit and reflects primarily water loss.(29) Much of this inital water loss is due to a poorly understood diuretic effect that occurs with sodium and water loss. The rest is the obligatory water loss that accompanies the depletion of glycogen stores. Later in a caloric-restriction diet, the diuresis stops entirely and in some instances a water gain can occur while net losses of fat and protein continue.

It is of interest to note that different diets can produce an accleration of weight loss due to greater water loss. For instance, a diet low in carbohydrate (the extreme is fasting) will cause greater diuresis and more precipitous weight loss. During a prolonged, partial or total caloric restriction, the body gradually adapts by conserving protein and water and increasingly burning fat to make up the energy deficit. Studies show that obese individuals accomplish this adaptation more rapidly than lean people.(29) However, the key finding is that *the body's fat loss is entirely proportional to its energy deficit.*

So, in the end, the type of diet is relatively unimportant for weight loss. What ultimately determines the loss is the degree of caloric deprivation. Because of this, most nutritionists now recommend a balanced diet that combines smaller portions of the basic foods with a drastic reduction or elimination of refined sugars and starches. Such a diet not only accomplishes weight reduction, but also establishes eating habits that promote the maintenance of desirable weight.

As surely as the sun rises and sets, there will always be one more diet which promises quick weight loss without effort. One fad that received a great deal of notoriety is "The Last Chance Diet" or "Protein-Supplemented Fasting," an essentially no-carbohydrate diet which supplies nutrition by a mixture of liquid proteins, vitamins, and minerals. The promoters of "The Last Chance Diet" claim that, when protein is provided in the diet, the body does not use its own protein, and thus minimizes muscle waste and the depletion of protein stores. But is this really so?

Not according to *New England Journal of Medicine*, which recently reported that, "Although some consider a low-calorie diet consisting entirely of protein to be uniquely advantageous in preserving body nitrogen, it has yet to be demonstrated convincingly that protein alone is more effective in this regard than an isocaloric mixture of protein and carbohydrate."(29) Indeed, this low-carbohydrate diet appears to be almost as bad as the Atkin's diet fad of a few years ago.

Whenever carbohydrate intake is severely restricted, as it is in the "The Last Chance Diet," fat is mobilized; the rapid mobilization of fat may cause serious side effects including liver damage. Dangerously low potassium levels may result, and even cardiac arrhythmia deaths have been attributed to this diet. The chemical imbalance created by the loss of salt, water, and other minerals may lead to weakness, faintness, and other side effects. What's more, because these diets do not encourage proper eating patterns, only one-third of those who follow them are able to keep fat off eighteen months after the weight loss.

The facts speak too clearly to be ignored: regardless of the current diet fads, if you eat too few calories too long, you will experience unhealthy changes in body function. The crux of sensible dieting is knowing what to eat and using a balanced diet that effects weight loss grad-ually.

Finally, a sensible exercise program will complement and contribute to proper weight loss. Several studies indicate that you can help prevent protein or muscle loss while dieting, by engaging in regular exercise. The key, then, to long-term prevention of obesity as well as to a total fitness program is learning how to eat and exercise properly, and doing it. With proper diet and proper exercise, you can expect to stay slim, vigorous, and healthy for years to come.

INFLUENCE OF DIET AND EXERCISE ON CHOLESTEROL, CARDIOVASCULAR DISEASE, AND ATHEROSCLEROSIS

The knowledge acquired over the past few decades about cholesterol, cardiovascular disease, and atherosclerosis indicates that a carefully combined program of diet and exercise can greatly retard these diseases. Arteriosclerosis is a process by which the walls of our body's blood vessels become infiltrated with fat that, in time, calcifies and forms plaques that can occlude an artery. It is seldom localized. When it develops in a major vessel to the brain or lower extremities, for example, there is nearly always similar impairment of the coronary arteries of the heart. In fact, the major cause of death in patients following surgery for localized atherosclerosis is heart attack.(6)

The precise mechanism by which cholesterol is deposited in the walls of arteries and an advanced plaque evolves is still being studied. It is apparent, though, that multiple defects in the cells' cholesterol metabolism are involved.

Our blood contains two classes of fats that are essential to life: cholesterol and triglycerides. Elevated levels of cholesterol and/or triglycerides are associated with accelerated atherosclerosis and increased probability of heart attack. Of the multiple factors that influence the blood levels of these fats, *diet, heredity,* and *exercise* are the most important. A reduction in blood triglyceride and cholesterol occurs with exercise and with a diet low in saturated fats.

Cholesterol is transported by protein compounds called *lipoproteins.* Recent investigations have shown that the *total level* of cholesterol is of less importance than the *ratio of high density lipoprotein (HDL)* to *low density lipoprotein (LDL).* Low density lipoproteins are the harmful transport vehicle that carries cholesterol into the tissues and enhances the build-up of fatty atherosclerotic plaques. Conversely, high density lipoproteins are capable of transporting cholesterol out of our arteries and tissues and into the liver where it is broken down and eliminated.

A high level of HDL to LDL correlates with a low risk for atherosclerosis and heart disease. Vigorous sustained exercise will raise high density lipoprotein levels and lower low density lipoprotein levels. A diet low in saturated fats will achieve the same result. Triglycerides are also lowered by exercise, and they correlate with the HDL to LDL ratio. Elevated triglyceride levels are seen with increased levels of low density lipoprotein while normal or low triglyceride levels are seen with elevated density lipoprotein levels.

Coffee, Alcohol, and Physical Exercise

A question that inevitably arises in the minds of those involved in a total exercise program is, "Must I stop drinking coffee and alcohol?" There is much misinformation about the effects of these two drugs. Several reports, for example, have suggested that moderate to heavy coffee drinking (6–10 cups daily) may predispose one to heart attack. More recent studies, however, show that coffee ingestion by itself is not harmful.(31) These earlier reports failed to account for the fact that many coffee drinkers are also cigarette smokers, a practice that does predispose one to heart attack, emphysema, and cancer. When cigarette smoking was taken into account, no increased incidence of heart attack was found in coffee drinkers.

Also contrary to earlier investigations, scientists now believe that moderate alcohol consumption, especially beer, is not harmful and indeed, appears to protect the heart. One study which covered a six-year period reported that "moderate beer drinkers" had only half the incidence of heart attack as those who totally abstained.(31) It is still unclear whether alcohol itself has some protective value, or whether the teetotaler represents a rigid personality type that may be predisposed to heart attack.

Beer has long been a favorite drink for many distance runners, and it is now often used as a replacement solution during long distance runs, including marathons. Indeed, beer has been credited with keeping the kidneys functioning during endurance exercise by blocking *antidiuretic hormone (ADH)* secretion and, thus, preventing kidney stones and hematuria from bruising of the bladder. It also has a high potassium and sodium ratio (5:1), and is a safe sweat replacement preventing *hypokalemia,* or low blood potassium. Beer also replaces *silicon,* an abundant non metallic element, and raises your high density lipoproteins. While there is no proof of improved performance from beer drinkers, it does appear that some of the discomfort in distance running may be alleviated.

One caution concerning alcohol consumption is its high caloric content of 7 calories per gram. Only fat, with 9 calories per gram, has more calories (protein and carbohydrates each contain only 4 calories per gram). Anyone dieting should be informed about the high caloric content of alcohol, and avoid or restrict its use.

All of us should be aware that excessive alcohol intake may cause direct toxic damage to the liver and in some cases to the heart as well. This is true even with an adequate diet. The old belief that cirrhosis of the liver develops primarily in people who drink heavily and eat poorly is myth, not fact. [Recent studies show that an average—size person who drinks one-half a bottle of 86 proof liquor per day for 25 years, has a 50 percent chance to develop cirrhosis of the liver regardless of the diet.] Today, in the United States, there are an estimated 10 million alcoholics, and in urban areas cirrhosis of the liver is the third major cause of death between the ages of 25 and 65 years. Therefore, while moderate alcohol consumption, especially beer, is certainly not harmful and may even protect the heart, heavy drinking is *very hazardous* and poisons the brain, heart, and liver.

VITAMINS: FACTS, FANCYS, AND MYTHS

For those of us following a strenuous, daily exercise program, a knowledge of vitamins is absolutely essential since we may need special vitamin supplements to achieve maximum benefit from our exercise.

No human, indeed no mammal, can function adequately on an exclusive diet of protein, carbohydrate, fat, and minerals. Additional factors present in natural, whole foods are required in minute amounts. These organic substances, called vitamins, function as chemical regulators

Table 2–1
Recommended Daily Allowances of Vitamins (United States)

Vitamin	Infants and Children < 4 yr	Children > 4 yr and Adults
Vitamin A	2,500 IU	5,000 IU
Thiamine (B_1)	0.7 mg	1.5 mg
Riboflavin (B_2)	0.8 mg	1.7 mg
Vitamin B_6	0.7 mg	2 mg
Vitamin B_{12}	3 mg	6 mg
Folic acid	0.2 mg	0.4 mg
Biotin	0.15 mg	0.3 mg
Niacin	9 mg	20 mg
Pantothenic acid	5 mg	10 mg
Ascorbic acid (C)	40 mg	60 mg
Vitamin D	400 IU	400 IU
Vitamin E	10 IU	30 IU

and are necessary for growth and the maintenance of life. There are fourteen known vitamins and they are divided into two basic groups: the fat-soluble vitamins, A, D, E, and K, and the water-soluble vitamins, C and the B-complex vitamins. Normally, a varied diet contains more than enough of these essential vitamins. But, because they do not contribute to body structure and are not a direct source of body energy, even the most active athlete needs little more than the sedentary person.

It has only been since the advent of the industrial revolution, urbanization, and sea travel, that many people have not had access to a varied farm diet of recently harvested foodstuffs, and that vitamin deficiencies have appeared. Sailors who spent months at sea without fruit or green vegetables, developed scurvy from a lack of vitamin C; impoverished Southeast Asians, who restricted their diets to polished rice, developed vitamin B deficiencies; and infants in crowded European slums, deprived of adequate sunlight, developed rickets from a deficiency of vitamin D.

One man who has contributed much to our understanding of vitamin deficiency is Professor Victor Herbert. Professor Herbert of Columbia University, College of Physicians and Surgeons, states succinctly that, "The sole unequivocal indication for vitamin therapy is vitamin deficiency." He discusses six ways in which vitamin deficiency develops: inadequate ingestion, absorption, or utilization; increased destruction, excretion, or increased requirement.(8) Of the six possible causes of vitamin deficiency that Herbert cites, inadequate ingestion is the only indication for dietary vitamin supplementation.

The fat-soluble vitamins (A, D, E, and K) are stored in the liver and adipose (fat) tissue. Deficiencies develop only after months or years of inadequate intake, and excessive intake will cause accumulated levels that can produce toxic side effects. The water-soluble vitamins (C and B—complex), are not stored in the body and must be constantly replenished in the diet. Deficiencies can develop in weeks, and when excessive amounts are ingested, the excess is excreted in the urine avoiding toxic accumulations.

Except during periods of extra—nutrient demand such as pregnancy, lactation, or prolonged illness, the AMA does not recommend vitamin supplementation. Today, however, the use of multivitamin preparations is commonplace. This is not harmful so long as fat-soluble vitamins are not taken in excess. However, the essential nutrients can come from our diet and need not be found in any vitamin bottle. These essential nutrients, i.e. those which cannot be manufactured by the body, include water, sources of energy (primarily carbohydrates), nine amino acids (building blocks of proteins), one fatty acid, a number of mineral elements, and vitamins. Only a diet including a selection from a wide variety of foods will insure adequate, essential nutrient intake.

Vitamins in Deficiency States

The American Medical Association advises that the use of vitamin preparations as dietary supplements ought to be restricted to specific instances of deficiency; and then only the deficient vitamins in therapeutic amounts prescribed along with measures to correct any dietary inadequacies. Some common medical conditions requiring vitamin therapy include the malabsorption syndromes (Tropical Sprue and Celiac Disease) where vitamins A,D,E, and K may be required. Therapeutic amounts of folic acid and/or B12 are needed in specific deficiency states including Pernicious Anemia. Pathological conditions of the intestines that require bowel resection or intestinal bypass will require vitamin therapy, the specific needs being dictated by the location of the bowel resection. In burn victims with extensive wounds to heal, vitamin C along with the B vitamins are frequently prescribed.

Thus a number of specific deficiency states do require vitamin therapy. To date, though, no conclusive evidence has been found to indicate that multivitamin preparations or megavitamin dosages have ever helped a patient. In fact, critical research is immediately needed to be certain that no harmful effects are being sustained by such practices. The toxic effects of excessive intake of vitamins A,D, and folic acid are known, and thus the Federal Drug Administration restricts the amounts of these vitamins available over the counter. The question remains unanswered; however, regarding the possible harmful effects of prolonged megavitamin doses of any of the other vitamins.

The Vitamin C Controversy

No vitamin has a more notable past or controversial present than Vitamin C. This vitamin, which occurs naturally in citrus fruits such as oranges, lemons, and limes, was first recognized by James Lind, a physician in the eighteenth-century British Navy, who linked its deficiency with scurvy, the dreaded sailor's disease. During the era of the great sailing ships, sailors deprived of fresh fruit and vegetables for months on end, developed scurvy, manifested by fatigue, easy bruising of the skin, and bleeding from the gums and mucous membranes. The scourge of the British Navy two hundred years ago, this disease was greatly relieved by the discovery that fresh fruit would prevent it. (The British sailors' use of limes earned them the nickname "Limeys.") Although the protective value of limes was discovered in the seventeen hundreds, the specific protective agent in the lime was not identified as Vitamin C until 1932.

Today, Vitamin C is in the news again because the Nobel Prize winning scientist Dr. Linus Pauling has proclaimed that large doses of Vitamin C aid the body's defense mechanisms against infection. Controversy rages, but no conclusive proof exists that Vitamin C in megadosages protects against the common cold or any other infection.

While the average non-exercising person may not need to supplement his diet with Vitamin C, it has been shown that people who engage in high levels of physical stress, or consume large quantities of alcohol, deplete the body's stores of Vitamin C. Smoking and even chewing tobacco, if the tobacco juice is swallowed, also lowers Vitamin C levels.(16) A diet high in char—broiled beef contains cholesterol oxide, a powerful oxidizer or substance that promotes the combination with oxygen with the resultant rapid depletion of both Vitamin C and E.

Our bodies cannot manufacture Vitamin C; it must be ingested. Thus, it isn't surprising that most athletes involved in endurance sports take supplements of Vitamin C in amounts from 500 mg, to 1 gram per day. A recent poll of members of the American Medical Joggers Association who were preparing for the Boston Marathon, revealed that over 90 percent of them took Vitamin C as a supplement. While no scientific proof of its effectiveness exists, many trainers and endurance athletes feel that supplemental Vitamin C greatly reduces the incidence of muscle and tendon injuries.

Vitamin C has also been implicated in the pathogenesis of atherosclerosis. A deficiency of Vitamin C may allow the lining of our arteries (the endothelium) to degenerate and form sites for arteriosclerotic deposits. From a medical standpoint, no harm is done, since excess Vitamin C that the body cannot use is promptly excreted in the urine. Indeed, for the vigorously exercising individual, 500 mg. to 1 gram of Vitamin C per day may well be beneficial. However, I must caution that ingestion of more than 4 grams per day has been associated with kidney stones, thus massive amounts are distinctly discouraged.

Cholesterol, Homocysteine, Vitamin B6, and Atherosclerosis

Currently, one of the most hotly contested scientific debates involves the homocysteine theory and the role of vitamin B6 in the prevention of atherosclerosis. *Homocysteine* is a toxic substance regularly produced from *methionine,* one of the amino acids in all the protein foods we eat. Since the body does not manufacture methionine, we must obtain it from dietary sources.

Normally, homocysteine is quickly converted to *cystathionine,* a non-toxic substance used in other biochemical reactions. Vitamin B6 acts as a co-enzyme or facilitator of the enzyme reaction that converts homocysteine to cystathionine. A deficiency of Vitamin B6 leads to a reduction in the cystathionine conversion, a buildup of homocysteine in the blood, and the appearance of an oxidized form, homocystine, in the urine.

Dr. Kilmer McCully, a professor of pathology at Harvard Medical School, is generally credited with suggesting homocysteine is the cause of atherosclerosis. He proposed in 1969 that too little vitamin B6 would retard the conversion of homocysteine to cystathionine, lead to elevated

Table 2–2
Relative B₆ and Protein Content of Foods

Food	mg B_6 (per 100 gm)	mg Methionine (per 100 gm)	Ratio of B_6 to Meth. ($\times$ 1000)	Standard Portion
Apple	.03	4	7.5	150 gms
Avocado	.42	19	22	123 gms
Banana	.51	11	46	150 gms
Beans, raw snap	.08	28	2.9	125 gms; 1 cup
Beef, raw round	.50	970	0.5	85 gms; 3 oz.
Bread, white	.04	126	0.3	23 gms; 1 slice
Bread, whole wheat	.18	161	1.1	23 gms; 1 slice
Broccoli, raw	.19	54	3.6	150 gms; 1 cup
Butter	.003	21	0.1	7 gms; 1 pat
Carrots	.15	10	15	50 gms
Cheese, cheddar	.07	653	0.1	17 gms; 1 in. cube
Chicken	.5	537	0.9	76 gms; ½ breast
Egg, hard-cooked	.11	392	0.3	50 gms
Lettuce, head	.07	4	17	220 gms; 4 in. head
Milk, cow whole	.042	83	0.5	244 gms; 1 cup
Oranges	.06	2.7	22	210 gms; 3 in. dia.
Peanut butter	.33	265	1.2	16 gms; 1 Tbs.
Peas, raw	.18	44	4.1	160 gms; 1 cup
Potato, raw	.25	25	10	100 gms
Spinach, raw	.28	54	5.2	180 gms
Tomato, raw	.10	8	12.5	150 gms
Yoghart, plain	.032	102	0.3	246 gms; 1 cup

blood levels of homocysteine, and thus promote atherosclerosis. Implicit in this theory were several predictions as
well as explanations of findings:

1. Humans and experimental animals eating vitamin B6
    —deficient diets should build up homocysteine in their
    blood.
2. If homocysteine is maintained in the blood of experi-
    mental animals, atherosclerosis should develop.
3. People proven to have atherosclerosis, such as coro-
    nary patients, ought to show a tendency toward low
    vitamin B6 in their blood.

In the last decade, each of these postulates has been
found to be true, and thus the theory is gaining momen-
tum. While a precise explanation of how homocysteine
exerts its effects remains a mystery, the theory is alive and
well, holding up nicely to its challengers.

Vitamin B6 is plentiful in fruits and vegetables, less so,
in meats and dairy products. At a glance, it would seem
unlikely that many people would be deficient in Vitamin
B6. It must be realized, though, that 80 to 90 percent of
Vitamin B6 is lost in milling wheat to produce white flour.
By cooking vegetables, you destroy two-thirds of their Vitamin B6 content, and cooking meat destroys 45 percent of
the vitamin. Therefore, it's no surprise that there are studies showing that most Americans eating "normal" diets do
not have adequate levels of Vitamin B6. This has been
found to be even more predominant in older Americans.

The homocysteine theory suggests most Americans eat
too much protein and refined starches, and not enough
fruit and vegetables——Vitamin B6 foods. It appears that
new criteria for food selection are on the horizon, not just
based on cholesterol, but on the relative B6 and protein
content (see Table 2-2).

While 2 mg./day of Vitamin B6 is currently considered
to be an adequate amount, many Americans eat less than

that, and there is considerable evidence to suggest that this level is too low to safely cover the entire adult population. Clearly, those groups prone to Vitamin B6 deficiency i.e., pregnant and nursing mothers, women on the contraceptive pill, dieters—especially those on a high protein regimen—and the elderly should receive more than 2 mg./day. Present evidence suggests that 10 mg./day of Vitamin B6 would provide a more appropriate margin of safety. This dosage would require supplements, because it would fit easily in a normal diet. Such levels are quite safe because excess Vitamin B6 is rapidly excreted and the toxic dose of the vitamin is more than 1,000 times greater than 10 mg./day.

A great deal remains to be learned about homocysteine. Conclusive proof of the theory awaits not only a molecular understanding of its action on the cells of blood vessels, but also, conclusive results from large-scale clinical testing over a number of years. Still, with the cholesterol theory experiencing a renewed challenge, and with inadequate explanations of all the aspects of atherosclerosis, the homocysteine theory deserves serious consideration. It is suggested that a lower intake of protein and a higher amount of Vitamin B6 may be desirable. Indeed, even in following a low-cholesterol diet, it would be helpful to lower protein intake.

Is the Cholesterol Theory in Trouble?

In a recent *New England Journal of Medicine,* Dr. George Mann, of Vanderbilt University Medical School, wrote:

A generation of research on the diet-heart question has ended in disarray. The official line since 1950 for management of the epidemic of coronary heart disease has been a dietary treatment. Foundations, scientists, and the media, both lay and scientific, have promoted low fat, low cholesterol polyunsaturated diets, and the epidemic continues unabated, cholesterolemia in the population is unchanged, and clinicians are unconvinced of efficacy.... This litany of failures must lead the clinician to wonder where the proper research and solutions lie. The problem of coronary heart disease is real enough here, and yet it is rare in less developed societies. What aspect of life-style here makes atherosclerosis so malignant, its clinical consequences so fearsome?(18)

This highly controversial paper sparked an almost unprecedented flood of letters to the editor. Certainly, the cholesterol hypothesis still claims the majority of physicians as supporters, but many have retreated to a position in which dietary cholesterol is only one of the more prominent of several risk factors in atherosclerosis.

The cholesterol theory can be traced to a Russian, I. A. Ignatovski, who, in 1808, was the first to demonstrate experimentally that, in rabbits, a high protein, high fat, high cholesterol diet rapidly caused arteriosclerosis. His results were quickly confirmed, but his assumption that protein played a major role was never accepted. When Anitschkow and Chalatow in 1813 produced rapid arteriosclerosis in rabbits by feeding them high cholesterol diets alone, the basic theory that high dietary cholesterol causes atherosclerosis was off and winging and has been popular ever since. It made no difference that others later showed feeding rabbits little or no cholesterol, but high protein diets, produced atherosclerosis even more rapidly; the cholesterol theory remained in popular acceptance.

Why is the cholesterol theory being re-evaluated in 1979? The answer lies in the fact that several very large, lengthy studies, one at the Mayo Clinic and the other at the National Institutes of Health sponsored Framingham study, both found little detectable relationship between diet cholesterol and serum cholesterol for people on a "normal" daily diet. That is, cholesterol in the diet didn't correlate with cholesterol blood levels.

This actually shouldn't come as a great surprise, as cholesterol is not a foreign substance; most is synthesized by the body itself rather than derived from dietary sources. Our bodies will manufacture up to 1,800 milligrams of cholesterol daily if none is eaten, and the amount our bodies produce drops as the amount we ingest increases. Thus, on a normal diet, one's cholesterol level may be higher or lower depending on other factors: exercise, smoking, genetics, fiber in diet, etc.

Even more important, regarding atherosclerosis, is that, a diet low in cholesterol or including cholesterol-lowering products such as fiber and yoghurt, results in only a 10 to 15 percent reduction in serum cholesterol. Is this really significant?

The serum cholesterol levels in Americans are 100 to 200 percent higher than the serum cholesterol levels of New Guinean highlanders in whom atherosclerosis is rare. So the small 10 to 15 percent reduction in serum cholesterol associated with even the strictest diets does not seem to make a major impact on the rate of atherosclerosis.

DIETARY FIBER—IS TODAY'S DIET DEFICIENT?

The most significant food sources of fiber are unprocessed wheat bran, unrefined cereals, and whole wheat and rye flours. Additional sources include fresh and dried fruit, raw vegetables, and legumes. It appears that of all the sources, wheat bran (the covering of the whole grain) is the most effective in increasing fecal bulk. This has led to commerical products of wheat bran on the grocery shelf with recommendations to add 6 teaspoons daily to everything from soup to chiffon cake.

Why is fiber important in our diet? Like many aspects of nutrition, there are both facts and unproven speculations. First, let's review the hard data. Fiber adds bulk to one's diet. Because most sources of fiber are relatively low in calories, this means you feel full while you have consumed fewer calories. The increased bulk facilitates transit time in your digestive tract. In one study, the transit time, duration from ingestion to anal elimination, decreased from 48 hours to 12 hours when the same subjects switched from a low to high fiber diet.(1)

A high fiber diet also produces stools that are softer, more bulky, and more frequent——on the average, one bowel movement every nineteen hours, containing twice as much carbohydrate, fat, and protein than those from an average diet. The increases in dietary fiber or "roughage," which increases fecal nutrient loss, have been calculated as energy losses that could account for an 8 to 10 pound *weight* loss over a one-year period.(1) Thus, a diet high in fiber, aids in weight control or reduction in two ways: first, it not only allows one to feel full with fewer calories consumed, but also affords a greater fecal loss of calories. There is a double reduction in caloric uptake by the body, one at each end so to speak!

A high fiber diet has been found to lower blood cholesterol too. (21) Because investigative reports are conflicting, it seems that the mechanism by which dietary fiber lowers cholesterol is unknown. That it occurs, however, raises speculation that the amount of fiber in the diet may be a factor in the prevention of atherosclerosis.

Whether there is any proven preventive disease benefit or not, most Americans do need to increase the fiber content of their diets to achieve the known beneficial effects discussed. Some may wish to sprinkle bran on various foods or substitute one-fifth bran for an equal part of flour in any baked foods; a significant increase in dietary fiber is most simply achieved by adding unprocessed cereals, whole wheat bread, salads, and some fresh or processed fruit on a regular basis.

Unproven Provocative Theories Regarding High Fiber Diets

The intake of crude fiber in the American diet has dropped 28 percent since the turn of the century. (9) While the intake of fiber from vegetables has remained relatively constant, consumption of potatoes, fruit, cereals, dry peas, and beans has declined. Coincident with this reduction of dietary fiber, has been an increase in a host of ailments including coronary heart disease, cholesterol gall stones, diabetes, obesity, hiatal hernia, peptic ulcer, constipation, diverticulosis, hemorrhoids, varicose veins, and cancer of the colon, all of which have been linked to *over*consumption of sucrose and highly milled starches and *under*consumption of fibrous materials in the diet. While most of the postulates remain controversial and inconclusive and are based on epidemiologic realtionships (populations with high fiber diets who have a low incidence of these problems), it is still interesting to review the physiological effects of fiber in the diet that relate to cause and effect or symptoms of these diseases and syndromes.

Fiber, by adding bulk to the feces, will eliminate constipation and render diverticulosis asymptomatic in seventy percent of the population. To the extent the stool is soft and one does not have to strain, the problem of hemorrhoids is lessened. As previously discussed, obesity can be combatted by a high fiber diet and its control affords a reduction in adult—onset diabetes and problems of varicosities. The anti-obesity and cholesterol lowering effect of fiber are both cited to explain its beneficient effect on heart disease. Furthermore, the cholesterol lowering effect accounts for the alleviation of cholesterol gall stones.

The increased transit time of feces may be a factor in reducing the occurrence of hiatus hernia, ulcer, and, most important, cancer of the colon. In the last half—century, while the fiber consumption from fruits and vegetables has declined by 20 percent, and from cereals and grain 50 percent, the incidence of cancer of the colon has risen significantly. Although unproven, much speculation exists that, by increasing the transit time through the colon threefold, the carcinogen or cancer—provoking agent—be it a virus or food breakdown product—is exposed to the large bowel for a much shorter period of time. It, therefore, has less opportunity to break down the natural resistance of the colon and produce cancer.

DIETARY REQUIREMENTS FOR THE VIGOROUSLY EXERCISING ADULT

The basic dietary need for the athlete or vigorously exercising adult is increased caloric intake. This means larger servings of foods, particularly carbohydrates, such as cereals, grains, and natural sugars in fresh fruit. Energy is provided less efficiently by fats, which should be polyunsaturated—derived from vegetable, nut, or seed sources, such as corn, safflower, and olives. Energy is provided least efficiently by protein. As indicated previously, the vitamin, mineral, and protein needs of most athletes are little different from sedentary spectators.

Besides larger food requirements, the person who exercises strenuously also has an increased need for water. The amount depends upon air temperature and on the intensity and duration of exercise. While fluid should be replaced during vigorous exercise, you must take note that the intestinal tract absorbs water at a significant rate of about 60 cc per hour. Thus, if perspiring freely, one cannot keep up with the water loss simply by replacing fluids. For this reason, endurance athletes such as marathon runners, who know they will lose four to eight pounds of water during a marathon, spend the hours immediately before the race drinking fluids until their urine is clear; they temporarily overload until the body excretes no "used" fluids. They actually start the race with several extra pounds of water in their bodies that will quickly be lost during the race. Likewise, the vigorously exercising adult should precede his or her workout by drinking fluids. Remember that thirst is not immediately sensitive to serious body dehydration—you may need fluids before you experience thirst. Therefore, plan increased fluid consumption based upon anticipated fluid losses.

Roughly 60 percent of the adult's body weight is water. If one's daily weight fluctuates by more than two pounds, fluid has not been adequately replaced. Such a significant water deficit will compromise physical performance and even threaten physical well being. Also, beverages containing caffeine (coffee, tea, cola, cocoa), as well as diets high in protein will increase urine production and even further deplete body fluids.

Salt Requirements

Too much has been made of the fact that we lose salt when we perspire. Actually, well-conditioned athletes lose only trace amounts of salt in their sweat. Habitual exercisers should not be concerned about salt needs as long as their diets are well rounded. Salt is ubiquitous in processed foods and *overly* plentiful in most diets—without ever reaching for the salt shaker. For most people, three daily meals easily replace the salt lost in up to ten pounds of exercise-induced sweat.

The Pre-exercise Meal

The pre-exercise meal serves the following needs: it minimizes hunger and weakness, ensures adequate hydration, provides for prompt emptying of the gastrointestinal tract, and protects against stomach upset. However, the traditional pre-game steak dinner is not recommended as a desirable nutritional preparation for vigorous exercise. The poorest source of energy, protein, compromises hydration by increasing urine output, and the fat in meat delays emptying of the stomach and upper gastrointestinal tract, promoting nausea and, in some instances vomiting.

Carbohydrates best support the glycogen and glucose stores needed for immediate energy and adequate blood sugar levels. Carbohydrate rapidly empties from the stomach and does not produce urinary diuresis. Therefore, the best pre-exercise diet should include modest amounts of high—carbohydrate foods taken at regular intervals with water or juices, up to two-and-a-half hours before exercise. In the immediate two-and-a-half hours preceding vigorous exercise, it is best to consume no solid foods [but clear fluids may be consumed.]

3

An Exercise Program
for the Obese

Imprisoned in every fat man a thin one is wildly signaling to
be let out

Cyril Connolly (1903–1974)

$\mathcal{A}$nyone seriously committed to a total physical fitness
program must also strive to achieve at least near optimum
body weight. In the United States, obesity statistics rise
rapidly at age 25, and by the fifth decade of life, one-third
of American men and over half of our women are more
than 20 percent overweight (obese). Unlike the days of the
flemish painter Rubens, today's society views obesity as
distinctly undesirable. Since the turn of the century, slen-
derness has been the ideal.

Most Americans now believe obesity is the number one
nutrition problem, a condition of "caloric excess." People
don't like to be fat. They dislike the unattractive appearance, general discomfort, and social stigma of obesity. The
concept of the "jolly" fat man or woman is pure myth. In

fact, hostility has been shown to be a key behavior reaction among the obese in recent psychological studies. (16) Most obese people agonize over walking appreciable distances, getting into a small car, or even buying clothes.

Over fifty million Americans spend over 100 million dollars annually for a quick easy way to lose weight. If one includes dietetic foods, "fat farms," "health spas," appetite-suppressing drugs, special exercise equipment, and the numerous devices for alleged spot—fat loss, the monetary figure zooms to over ten billion dollars in the United States alone.(16)

To be obese places a severe strain on your body (even more so while exercising); that is why I have selected specific exercise programs for the obese. More important, obesity contributes directly to hypertension and adult-onset diabetes (70–80 percent of adult-onset diabetics are obese), and indirectly to heart disease and stroke.(8) Life insurance companies' statistics clearly show that the overall death rate of the obese adult is over fifty percent greater than that of the normal-weight adult of comparable age.

High blood pressure and obesity have both been identified as risk factors for coronary heart disease. Hypertension also increases the chance of stroke and accelerates the process of atherosclerosis. In the Framingham study, it was found that, as people gained weight, they experienced proportionally higher levels of blood pressure (hypertension) and cardiovascular disease. These patterns appeared in both sexes, but were more prominent in men. For example, middle-aged males 30 percent overweight were *four times* more likely to die suddenly of heart attack and *seven times* more likely to suffer a stroke than lean males of comparable age.(6)

While research like the Framingham study established a direct relationship between obesity and hypertention during the past ten years (3, 6, 7, 15), many other studies have shown the converse, namely that a fall in blood pressure can be expected with a reduction in weight.(3,7) The same Framingham study found that a 15 percent weight loss in males, was associated with a 10 percent drop in blood pressure. In a recent study in the *New England Journal of Medicine*, similar findings were reported for a group of hypertensive, obese females. The authors concluded that, "Weight control is a potent tool in the control of hypertension in overweight subjects."(14)

Since a sizable proportion of hypertensive patients are obese, weight control might complement drug treatment, reduce the required dose, or even obviate the need for it in a considerable part of the hypertensive population. Weight reduction should, therefore, be recommended as the initial step in the treatment of any hypertensive patient who is above ideal weight. (These researchers also established that a fall in blood pressure was not due to a reduction in salt intake, but instead was associated directly with a reduction in body fat.)

Obesity has also been linked to elevated blood cholesterol levels. However, the effect of obesity on blood pressure is considerably greater than on cholesterol. Obesity is dangerous primarily because it causes hypertension. Most physicians recommend caloric restriction as the treatment of choice for the mildly hypertensive, overweight patient. Actually, the best treatment is a combined one of exercise and diet, especially since tests have established that strenuous, regular exercise by itself usually results in some weight loss and a lowering of blood pressure.

Unfortunately, our understanding of the relationship between diet and exercise and a reduction in weight and blood pressure is still tentative. How obesity predisposes one to hypertension, for example, is as unclear as how it is associated with diabetes. Hopefully, in view of the great number of obese, hypertensive people in our society, the federal government will deal with this serious problem by making and funding an intensive research commitment in this area of health care.

WHAT CONSTITUTES OBESITY AND HOW IS IT MEASURED?

It is essential to realize that being overweight and being obese are not necessarily synonymous, even though in practical terms obese generally means more than 15–20 percent overweight. Realistically, obesity should be regarded as 15 percent or more excess body fat. Overweight refers to excess weight as compared with sex, height, and body-frame. It includes all body components: muscle, water, minerals, tissue, as well as fat. Thus, weight lifters and body builders who have markedly enhanced muscle development may be grossly "overweight," but may have no excess fat and thus, not be obese. The basic concept exists, then, that obesity refers only to body fat, the tissue accumulated exclusively by caloric excess.

Body fat can be measured by several techniques. One of the most accurate is the immersion technique of comparing body weight in air and under water. While valuable in the research laboratory, it is not practical for us at home. It is also not essential. The simplest test is a self-examination made before a mirror. A fat appearance denotes obvious obesity. The "ruler "test" may be used for those wanting to be more precise or those inclined to be more lenient in regard to what looks fat. With this test, again stripped, you lie on your side on a flat, firm surface such as the floor. Place a yardstick on the side facing up, from the rib cage to the pelvis. If the ruler can be passed flat, obesity is not present, while the presence of a rounded contour denotes obesity. Perhaps the easiest and most accurate way to assess obesity is by measuring multiple body skin folds. The triceps skin fold thickness behind our upper arm is representative of total body fat. Seltzer and Stare have suggested figures of 2.3 centimeters and 3.0 centimeters for male and female adults as minimums defining the presence of obesity. (11) A caliper calculated in millimeters is the only piece of equipment needed for this test. As body fat is lost, a proportionate reduction in the skin fold measurement is realized.

WHY WE BECOME OBESE AND HOW TO CORRECT IT

While rare hypothalamic, genetic, and drug-induced obesities do occur, almost all adult-onset obesity is simply due to the fact that more calories are consumed than are used by the body. Eliminating obesity requires decreasing caloric intake, increasing caloric expenditure, or preferably both, so that, until desirable weight is achieved, the body runs a daily deficit of calories and burns body fat to compensate.

As discussed in the nutrition chapter, over a long period of time, the composition of the diet—if nutritionally adequate—really doesn't matter, as long as there is a deficit of calories. While many studies have shown the most precipitous weight loss on a short-term diet occurs with a high-fat diet, next with a high-protein, and least a high-carbohydrate diet, the impressive, rapid drop in weight on the high-fat diet reflects water loss and not fat reduction. This is like jogging in a rubber suit to increase perspiration, rapidly deplete body water, and temporarily lose body weight. Given access to fluids, the depleted body water will quickly be replaced and only the true fat loss (a deficit of 3,500 calories equals one pound) will be reflected on the scales.

THE ANALOGY BETWEEN OBESITY AND DIABETES

It is now clear that overcoming obesity requires a reduction in caloric intake below caloric expenditure. The physician must (1) determine where the patient is out of caloric balance (overeating, inactivity, or both), (2) recognize the patient's "problem" times of the day and associated activities, (3) encourage small but well-reinforced changes that are likely to become permanent, such as extra walking (4) encourage no more than 1–2 pounds of weight loss per week which is 500 calories less per day, (5) discourage fad diets and emphasize a nutritious diet chosen from natural food preferences, (6) encourage slow eating with techniques like putting down utensils between mouthfuls and chewing well so the patient will feel full with less food.

In addition, there must be a lucid plan of weight maintenance once the desired weight is achieved. Most physicians now feel the weight maintenance phase should be simultaneous with the weight loss phase. It should be pictured as an ongoing process, because there are no known cures for adult onset obesity except caloric equilibrium. Here, there is the strong parallel with diabetes. In each illness, the physician accepts the responsibility for the initial diagnosis and treatment plan, but the ultimate day-to-day management of the condition is up to the patient. Whereas the weight loss phase is generally under the direction of the physician, the success of the weight maintenance phase rests with the patient. The physician must be successful in this shift of responsibility if long term maintenance of desired weight is to be achieved.

Inherent in weight maintenance, is education in a nutritionally adequate, appetite-satisfying, low—to—moderate calorie diet. While personal preferences must be taken into consideration, some general features include the following:

1. lean meat, fish, or fowl at least once daily, plus up to three eggs weekly;
2. unsweetened cereal or a slice of whole wheat bread two or three times daily;
3. green or yellow vegetables twice daily;
4. fruit or fruit juice twice daily;

5. at least 300 calories at each of three or four meals without snacking;
6. reasonable size portions without second servings;
7. broil, boil, bake, or roast meat and fish; remove visible fat, avoid thickened gravy;
8. cook vegetables without fat, flavor with vegetable margarine, herbs, or bouillon;
9. favor green, yellow, or red vegetables over starchy ones;
10. use low-calorie salad dressings, lemon juice, and/or vinegar;
11. plain fruit for dessert;
12. sweeten with sugar substitutes, use only sugar-free soft drinks;
13. eat meals at about the same time each day with regular intervals in between;
14. favor non-fat milk, ice milk, or low-fat ice cream;
15. minimize alcoholic beverages, use "lite" beers, have sugar-free soft drinks as mixes.

An Exercise Program Tailored to the Obese

While the obese can lose weight with a diet alone, weight reduction—and especially maintenance—is far easier and more successful with a simultaneous program of exercise. Exercise not only burns up calories, but it also can act as an appetite suppressant. Moderate exercise has been shown not to increase appetite, but rather, to have an anorexic effect. (5) An appropriate exercise program, while important for anyone because of the many physical and psychological benefits (see Table 1-1, page 34), acquires even more significance for the obese. This is because such a program combats the various risk factors of cardiovascular disease and stroke that obesity promotes: diabetes, hypertension, and hyperlipidemia.

An appropriate exercise program for the obese shares most of the same basic features as others: a warm-up period, an aerobic endurance phase, and a cooling-off period. The frequency of exercise should not be less than three days per week, and preferably more. Before it is begun, however, a medical examination with a stress electrocardiogram should be obtained, because of the greater risk of heart disease in the obese.

The warm-up and cooling-off periods should last five to ten minutes. Each involve rhythmic slow stretching movements of the trunk and limbs that emphasize a range of motion of joints. Carried out before vigorous exercise, these movements enhance blood flow, stretch and loosen one's muscles preparing them for sustained activity, and minimize the chance for strains or sprains. Following vigorous exertion, they faciliate the various bodily functions[3] gradual return to normal, and promote the elimination of waste products from your muscles, thereby lessening the possibility of stiffness or soreness the following day.

Calisthenics are ideal for each of these periods. In Table A–1, page 187 and Table A–3, page 188, specific exercises for each of these periods are listed. You may select any combination of three or more from each table to constitute your own warm-up and cooling-off period. It is recommended that you vary the selection of exercises on different days, both to avoid monotony as well as ensure total body involvement.

The most important portion of your exercise program in regard to weight reduction and all the other positive factors listed in Table 1–1, page 34, is the endurance phase. This phase should ideally involve activities that use the large muscle groups of the body in a continuous, rhythmic, aerobic manner. The duration should eventually exceed thirty minutes, although a more modest beginning may be necessary. As the training effect is realized and your aerobic capacity is enhanced, you may increase the intensity and duration of this period.

You should not, while excercising, exceed an intensity greater than 60 to 80 percent of your maximal oxygen uptake or heart rate (about 120–140 beats per minute); nor a duration of one hour. While competitive athletes must exceed these limits in order to achieve maximum performance, it is with a significantly increased risk of injury. This risk is undesirable for your exercise program; while enthusiasm is to be applauded, getting carried away is to be avoided.

In the upright position, the excess weight of obesity places greater stresses on your low back, hips, knees, ankles, and feet, both at rest and with exertion. The types of endurance exercises best suited for the obese, are therefore more restricted than for the slender. In Table 3–1 some of the better endurance exercises for the obese are listed. No jogging or running exercises are listed because the strain on the low back and lower extremities is too great. Multiple studies have shown an increased incidence of injury of up to 50 percent in the obese who are beginning a jogging program. (4, 6, 9) Clearly, activities involving running and jumping where obesity accentuates the vertical stresses to the musculoskeletal system are to be avoided.

While temporarily obese, the best exercises are those done in water, body surfing, scuba diving, skin diving, swimming, or water polo; those pursued in a sitting position i.e., bicycling, canoeing, kayaking, and rowing; or those done erect, without much running or jumping i.e., backpacking, boxing, cross-country skiing, handball, hiking, ice hockey, ice skating, karate, racquetball, roller skating, snowshoeing, squash, walking, and wrestling.

Swimming is the best all-around aerobic exercise for the obese, as all the major muscle groups receive vigorous exercise while the stesses to the skeletal system of the body are minimal and are actuallly made less by the increased body fat. Body fat adds to one's buoyancy in water and partially accounts for the fact that most great marathon swimmers are on the chubby side. Swimming is also rhythmic, by definition continuous, and of necessity aerobic. Thus, it meets all the criteria of a good endurance exercise without allowing the excess weight to stress one's skeletal system.

However, after you have shed weight by the combination of diet and your own exercise program, I encourage you to explore the additional exercises found in Chapters 8 and 9. Your obesity with a diligent approach will be quite temporary; and as you enter the weight maintenance phase that we all must pursue for the rest of our lives, only personal preferences need limit your choice of recreational pursuits.

Table 3–1

Aerobic Endurances Exercise Pursuits for the Obese

Backpacking	Paddleball
Bicycling	Racquetball
Body surfing	Roller skating
Boxing	Rowing
Canoeing	Scuba diving
Cross-country skiing	Skin diving
Handball	Snowshoeing
Hiking	Squash
Ice hockey	Swimming
Ice skating	Walking
Karate	Wrestling
Kayaking	Water polo

4

Exercise for the Diabetic

Better to hunt in fields, for health unbought, than fee the doctor for a nauseous draught. The wise, for cure, on exercise depend; God never made his work for man to mend.

John Dryden (1631–1700)

THE METABOLISM OF DIABETES

Diabetes is an inherited metabolic abnormality characterized by a relative or absolute lack of insulin secretion from a gland in the abdomen called the pancreas. Insulin is required to store glucose in our muscles and our liver. Glucose is the preferred fuel for the cells of our body and insulin is the hormone that allows the cells to take glucose from the blood and burn (metabolize) it. The presence of insulin also retards the burning of body fat. When food intake is denied, the body reacts to cell starvation by releasing very low levels of insulin. Initially, glucose is released from the liver, and later, when this source is depleted, free fatty acids are released from our fat stores as a fuel source for our body's cells. In a prolonged fast lasting days, even the protein in the muscles of the body is converted to a fuel source.

Diabetes can thus be compared to starvation of the cells of our body. With a lack of insulin, the cells cannot take glucose out of the blood and metabolize it. This means the blood level of glucose remains high (hyperglycemia). The cells, being unable to utilize glucose in the absence of insulin, burn fat as fuel. Thus, there are paradoxical findings of high blood sugar (hyperglycemia) and the products of starvation metabolism (high free fatty acids, cholesterol, and ketone bodies). The diabetic, burning his body fat, loses weight as the body cells are starved.

THE THREE STAGES OF DIABETES

Diabetes can be thought of as existing in three phases. Before the clinical form of overt diabetes occurs, two other stages, *prediabetes* and *chemical diabetes* exist.

Prediabetes exists from the time of conception, as diabetes is an inherited, genetic, disease. There are no signs or symptoms in the prediabetic state; all tests of carbohydrate tolerance are normal and no diabetic vascular complications occur. These individuals are normal in every way, yet we know the stage does exist. The diabetic gene is certainly present in all identical twins of diabetic parents. Yet the incidence of diabetes in such twins is only 50 percent. Half of the identical twins of diabetic parents never develop diabetes.

Chemical diabetes exists when tests of carbohydrate tolerance are abnormal. The most commonly used test is the oral glucose tolerance test. The patient goes without eating for 12 hours, empties his bladder, then consumes a sugar-rich drink. At 30 minute intervals during a 2 - 4 hour period, venous blood samples and urine specimens are taken. The normal response is one where all blood sugar values are well under 180 mg. % (180 mg. of sugar/100 ml of plasma), and no sugar is found in the urine. In the chemical and overt stages of diabetes, blood sugar levels readily exceed 180 mg. % and sugar is found in the urine.

In the chemical diabetic stage, the signs and symptoms of diabetes are absent and no medical treatment is indicated. Most agree, though, that these individuals are the ones most likely to develop overt diabetes, and they should be followed closely. In addition, they should adopt the lifestyle of the adult, non-insulin dependent diabetic i.e., dietary restriction of refined sugar, advoidance of obesity, and regluar daily exercise.

Overt diabetes is accompained by the triad of *polyuria* (frequent urination), *polydipsia* (thirst), and *polyphagia* (incessant hunger) all accompanied by weight loss. As explained earlier, the body's cells are literally being starved to death by the inability to use glucose, due to the lack of insulin. The most frequent precipitating causes of the change from chemical to overt diabetes are infection and emotional upset. However any prolonged stress, such as pregnancy, may be a precipitating factor. The overt, undetected diabetic feels weak and listless and, if not treated, will advance to coma and death.

Prior to the discovery of insulin in 1921 by Drs. Frederick Banting and Charles Best, juvenile diabetes and severe adult—onset diabetes were uniformly fatal. With the use of animal—derived insulin, diabetes, while not actually cured, can be largely controlled. The life expectancy for most adult-onset diabetics is little changed; for the childhood-onset diabetic, the statistics are not quite as favorable, due to vascular complications in older age.

The use of single or multiple daily injections of animal insulin, however, has allowed the diabetic to live a vigorous, essentially normal life through youth and middle age. Whereas formerly, many juvenile diabetics would have died before they could bear or produce children, the discovery of insulin meant their reproduction would be uneffected. As a consequence, this genetically transmitted disease is steadily increasing. In 1974 the National Committee on Diabetes was established, and it reported an incidence increase of over 50 percent between 1965 and 1973. Five percent of Americans now have diabetes and the current rate of increase is six percent per year. The number of Americans with diabetes, ten million, is projected as double that by 1990.(5)

In view of the millions of people involved, the economic impact of treating this disease is major. It is further magnified when we consider the complications seen in diabetics. In the last quarter-century, with the longer survival rate of diabetic patients, the vascular complications leading to blindness, kidney failure, nervous system disorders, and cardiovascular disease have become all too apparent. Although there is controversy, most feel these complications are accelerated by poor diabetic control and retarded by excellent control. *As of March 1976, the American Diabetes Association stated that a high level of metabolic control will prevent or delay microvascular disease.*

It is unfortunate that not until 1976 did Congress pass the *National Diabetes Act* which has allocated money for diabetes research and created a permanent advisory board to supervise the carrying out of the act.(13) Much research is required to resolve the questions regarding exactly what is optimal control. This is important not only from the standpoint of preventing vascular complications, but also, in preventing insulin reactions—a not uncommon occurrence when control too precise is attempted. Excessive control is not only harmful, but can be fatal. The low blood sugar caused by excessive insulin can lead to coma, with loss of brain cells, altered memory and mental capacity, as well as death.

To date, there has never been a study that relates long-term control to the development of diabetic complications because we have not had adequate measures of long—term control.(13) The assessment of diabetic control remains crude. The diabetic can measure his or her urine several times a day for the degree of sugar present; this is a rough estimate of the level of blood sugar presented to the kidneys several hours previously. However, since the threshold or level of blood sugar that will cause sugar to appear in the urine varies from person to person, the same level of blood sugar may cause 1+ urine glucose in one and 3+ in another.

A more accurate test can be done with Dextrostix, plastic sticks available from a drugstore, which measure blood glucose levels from a finger prick. While this is superior to the urine sugar measurement (using a Tes-Tape), it still gives only the blood level at a fixed moment out of 24 hours. It is also expensive—each stick costs about half a dollar. In addition, it is uncomfortable and few people are willing to carry it out routinely. We know that, even with insulin use, blood sugar levels fluctuate widely in diabetics. To assess the degree of control, we would, ideally, need to know the blood sugar level continuously throughout every day.

Recently, a new blood test has been devised that allows assessment of the level of blood glucose over a period of months. This test involves the measurement of a particular type of hemoglobin, the protein within the red blood cell that carries oxygen to and from the tissues. This hemoglobin molecule has a glucose molecule attached to one of its structural chains. The amount of this *glycostated hemoglobin* directly reflects the blood sugar level. As the blood sugar is elevated, more glucose is tied up with the hemoglobin and is present as long as the red cell is alive, about 120 days. This glycostated hemoglobin accurately reflects the average level of diabetes control over a period of 2 to 3 months.(13) Now, for the first time, studies relating the true degree of diabetic control and the development of diabetic complications are underway.

TESTS FOR THE EARLY DETECTION OF DIABETES

Most diabetologists agree that mass screening for diabetes in children is hardly worth the cost, as very few cases are detected and not all prediabetics or chemical diabetics will become overt diabetics. There are exceptions, when early diabetes detection is warranted: among the select population with a strong family history of the disease; children with sugar in their urine or with other symptoms of the disease; and obese children.

While the tests to be described later are more precise, the following is a simple test any mother can do at home. In the morning, before breakfast, have your child empty his bladder. Give the child over 6 years of age 8 ounces of orange juice with 1 tablespoon of sugar added. Follow this with a 12 ounce bottle of coke. Then 2–3 hours later, test your child's urine for sugar either with a *Clinitest* tablet or paper *Tes-Tape*. For the child under 6 years of age, use half the amount of orange juice, sugar, and coke. If the urine test is positive, the child should be taken to a diabetic medical specialist or a diabetes clinic for further evaluation.

In adults, diabetes is much more prevalent and the incidence rises sharply with advancing age. For this reason, most adults should be and are screened for diabetes with their annual physical examination, or when they are admitted to a hospital for any reason. The standard test is a blood sugar drawn 2 hours after a meal rich in carbohydrate. While not as precise as a glucose tolerance test, it suffices as a mass screening device. The adult can also test himself in the manner described previously for the child. Just follow the same sequence, but *double* the amount of orange juice, sugar, and coke. In addition to the tests described, exercise has provided a means for detecting the very early diabetic or diabetic-prone individual. During exercise, the diabetic has a marked rise in blood glycerol and free fatty acids. Statistically, the rise is significantly greater after 30 minutes of strenuous exercise and it remains elevated for another 40 minutes. This same type of glycerol and free fatty acid rise has been seen in some pre-diabetics,(28) causing researchers to speculate that, possibly 15 to 20 percent of the pre-diabetics who show the diabetic—type rise in glycerol and free fatty acids in response to exercise will eventually develop diabetes.(28) Studies are presently in progress to determine the validity of this hypothesis.

THE GENETICS OF JUVENILE-ONSET DIABETES MELLITUS

Dr. James V. Neel of the U.S. Public Health Service has recently called the genetics of diabetes mellitus the "geneticist's nightmare."(27) Evidence now suggests that stable, maturity-onset diabetes may have a different genetic background than the more unstable juvenile-onset diabetes. In fact, as will be discussed more fully under diet, considerable evidence indicates that most maturity-onset diabetes can be prevented by weight control. Why the genetic transmission of juvenile-onset diabetes remains a mystery is that the incidence of this disease in identical twins from diabetic parents is only 50 percent. Thus in genetically identical offspring only half contract juvenile diabetes mellitus.

A current, tentative explanation of this mystery is that a virus causes diabetes in genetically—prone individuals.(8, 9, 14) The theory suggests that, in some people born with the inherited tendency for diabetes, certain viral infections can destroy their insulin—secreting, pancreatic beta cells. In test animals there are many examples of specific viral infections causing destruction of the beta cells in a process similar to that in juvenile diabetes.

For the last five years, at Childrens Hospital in Boston, blood serum samples from all new diabetic patients have been collected and frozen to store until such viruses can be identified and studied. Whether the cause is viral or not, the chance of a child having diabetes is 25 percent when one parent has the disease and the other is normal, and 50 percent when both parents have it.

MUST INSULIN ALWAYS BE REFRIGERATED?

Every child with overt diabetes should be regulated on insulin as soon as the diagnosis is made. Oral hypoglycemic agents should not be given to children, because they do not control the disease, and, eventually, will only further deplete the pancreas. So, too, the lean, active adult who develops diabetes must be regulated on insulin.

One of the first things the diabetic learns, besides how to administer an injection, how much and often to take insulin, and how to recognize and treat an insulin reaction, is the notion that the insulin itself must be kept refrigerated. This poses an awkward and unnecessary problem for the diabetic. Unless one stays at home, the constant refrigeration of insulin is difficult—and frequently impossible—since most insulin diabetics require injections twice a day (a common practice is ⅔ of the total insulin requirement before breakfast and ⅓ before dinner).

In reality, one need not worry about the potency of the insulin unless it's frozen, which ruins it, or subjected to very high temperatures, which weakens it. If you are outside in the winter, skiing, simply keep it in a packet close to your body; when traveling in the heat, keep it out of the direct sun. Of course, when refrigeration is available, use it. But realize that insulin will retain its potency at room temperature for days, and sometimes, up to a year.

HOW TO CHOOSE YOUR DOCTOR

Before the diabetic begins as exercise program, he or she should undergo a thorough physical examination. If over 35, a stress electrocardiogram should be included in the check-up, because the diabetic is a risk for cardiovascular disease. Undoubtedly, most diabetics already have a doctor, but is he the one to prescribe your exercise program?

Obviously, the physician must be qualified. But there are some simple questions you can ask yourself that are likely to indicate when a second opinion is in order. Did your doctor ask you to curtail your physical activities when your diabetes was diagnosed? Did your doctor place any physical restrictions on your life? Is your doctor physically inactive himself? Is your doctor obese? Does your doctor smoke heavily? Does your doctor paint a bleak outlook for normal life? Does your doctor prescribe rigid insulin requirements and place none of the responsibility for management on you? Does your doctor seem distant and difficult to communicate with? If the answer to one or more of the above questions is yes, you probably have the wrong doctor for your diabetic management and exercise program.

Do not be apologetic or afraid to seek a second opinion; your life is at stake! Realize that no worthwhile, mature physician will ever be offended by a patient seeking a second opinion. And most doctors would prefer to have patients with whom they have little rapport cared for by other physicians. How do you find the right doctor? There are no absolute answers. In general you will do better with a specialist in diabetes who is himself in good physical condition, a sports enthusiast, and with whom you can establish a rapport.

THE METABOLISM OF EXERCISE

When the diabetic undertakes a regular daily regimen of 30–60 minutes of vigorous physical activity, it is a common occurrence that insulin requirements decrease—often as much as 50 percent—while carbohydrate intake may increase. In fact, many adult-onset diabetics no longer require insulin after starting an exercise program! To understand how exercise can accomplish this, we must first examine the metabolism of exercise in non-diabetics.

While fat and carbohydrate each contribute about 40 percent of the caloric content of the average American diet, the body stores fuel almost entirely in the form of fat (triglyceride stores in fatty tissue). The remainder of our immediate fuel stores is glucose (sugar) stored in our muscles and the liver as glycogen. During the earliest phase of muscular activity, the first 5–10 minutes, glucose stored in the muscles is the major fuel source. As exercise continues, glucose is released from the liver and muscle blood-flow, and glucose uptake rises 7–20 times the resting level (depending on the intensity of the exercise performed).(35)

Initially most of the glucose released from the liver is from *glycogenolysis,* the release of glucose already stored in the liver as glycogen. As the duration and intensity of exercise increases, a greater amount of liver glucose release occurs from the process of *gluconeogenesis,* the synthesis or manufacture of glucose. This is the sequence of fuel utilization in prolonged exercise: First the muscle burns glucose already stored in it, then glucose, primarily released from the liver, is taken from the blood stream, and finally the food source is free fatty acids from the body's fat stores.

When exercise stops, blood flow to muscles decreases, but the uptake of glucose remains 3–4 times the resting level for nearly an hour. This attempt to replenish glucose takes place in the liver, too, for even longer periods of time.(11) Insulin levels rise after exercise to facilitate this response.

However, *during exercise, insulin levels decrease, while muscle intake of glucose increases!* This indicates that, during exercise, the muscle intake of glucose does not require increased insulin. The exact mechanism by which exercising muscle can take glucose from the blood stream is not fully understood. Nevertheless, it is this very occurrence, that is, perhaps, primarily responsible for the reduced insulin requirements and improvement in glucose tolerance that is seen in diabetics who are exercising. Exercise, not only burns calories and lowers blood sugar, but it accomplishes that without insulin.

This does raise a potential problem for the insulin-dependent diabetic. The release of insulin from a subcutaneous injection is steady, and does not fall during exercise. In fact, if the lower extremities are used as the injection site, insulin release is speeded up by exercise. This means that the liver will not release glucose into the bloodstream in the way it will in the normal person who has a drop in insulin levels during exercise.

Glycogenolysis is reduced in the diabetic. This is partially offset by the fact that gluconeogenesis is enhanced. However, the net effect is reduced liver glucose output, so the insulin-dependent diabetic is potentially a risk for hypoglycemia or low blood sugar unless they either *decrease their intake of insulin, or increase their intake of carbohydrates* before engaging in unusually strenuous prolonged exercise.

Exercise, therefore, affords a reduction in insulin requirements and liberalization of carbohydrate intake in the insulin-dependent diabetic. For many adult-onset diabetics, it can eliminate insulin requirements entirely and return glucose tolerance to normal i.e., "cure" the disease.

Well-regulated diabetics have an exercise metabolism which is not different in principle from that of similarly trained non-diabetic subjects. This is true in both juvenile and adult-onset diabetics. Furthermore, moderate to severe exercise increases tolerance for glucose in both normal and diabetic males. (23) Since it is not mediated by insulin, as expected, it has been shown that glucose intake by exercising muscle is not reduced in diabetes. So, too, the cardiovascular adaptation to exercise is similar in diabetic and non-diabetic patients alike. (36)

The message for the diabetic is loud and clear. *Exercise is mandatory for maximal control of your disease, and daily exercise will very likely retard the development of vascular complications. Your cardiovascular system can become conditioned as quickly as the non—diabetic's. There is no exercise you should avoid. Your only risk factor is hypoglycemia, with sustained exercise over forty minutes, and your carbohydrate intake and/or insulin administration must be adjusted accordingly.* There are diabetics running marathons and actively pursuing many other competitive endurance sports (see Table 4–1).

Because of the long-term value of exercise for the diabetic, diabetic children should be taught and motivated to be physically active during their entire lives. Their parents and teachers should direct them into sports like running or swimming, that can be pursued through adulthood, that place sufficient stress on the cardiovascular system, and that can be done at any time with little cost. Since exercise will help to control their disease, diabetic children should learn that daily physical conditioning will stabilize both their insulin and diet requirements.

DIET, EXERCISE, AND DIABETES

In human beings, the two most important environmental factors related to the development of diabetes, appear to be inadequate physical activity and excessive calorie intake.

Recent studies have changed the dietary management and attitudes toward exercise in the prevention and treatment of diabetes and its complications.(4, 41) The new strategies for diabetic control are illustrated by the consideration of these practical questions: Can diet and exercise prevent diabetes? What are the purposes of diabetic diets? Are the vascular lesions of diabetes preventable? Is diet therapy feasible?

Table 4–1
Some Exercise Pursuits Carried Out by Diabetics

Archery	Gymnastics	Running
Backpacking	Handball	Sailing
Badminton	Hiking	Sailplanes
Baseball	Hockey	Scuba diving
Basketball	Horseback riding	Show jumping
Bicycling	Hunting	Skin diving
Boating	Ice fishing	Sky diving
Body building	Ice hockey	Snowshoeing
Body surfing	Ice skating	Soccer
Bowling	Isometrics	Softball
Boxing	Jogging	Spelunking
Calisthenics	Jumping rope	Sports car rallying
Camping	Karate	Squash
Canoeing	Kayaking	Surfing
Cross-country running	Lawn bowling	Swimming
Cross-country skiing	Motocross	Tennis
Dancing	Motorcycling	Tobogganing
Diving	Paddleball	Track
Downhill skiing	Ping-Pong	Tumbling
Field hockey	Platform tennis	Volleyball
Fishing	Pool	Walking
Folk dancing	Rock climbing	Waterskiing
Football	Rodeo	Weight lifting
Gliding	Roller skating	Wrestling
Golf	Rowing	

CAN DIET AND EXERCISE PREVENT DIABETES?

The answer is unquestionably yes, as the incidence of diabetes among different societies of the same race may differ as much as ten times the rate, depending on work and diet circumstances.(39, 42) While diabetes is common in some groups of whites, blacks, Indians, native Americans, Chinese, Japanese, Polynesians, and Jews, it is rare in other groups of the same ethnic background who eat and exercise differently.(39, 43) This suggests that, in a majority of adult cases, diabetes is preventable, and that the major predisposing factors are weight and exercise.

It is now evident that the risk of diabetes is greatly increased by excessive caloric intake—whether the calories come from fat, protein, or carbohydrates.(44) For example, the very fat sumo-wrestlers of Japan consume a diet high in starch and low in sugar. In this traditional Japanese sport, where the objective is to pin the opponent to the mat or toss him out of the ring, great body size and weight is an advantage. Large men are recruited and placed on diets ranging from 5,000 to 6,000 calories per day, 80 percent carbohydrate. Exercise is intense but brief, so no endurance cardiovascular improvement takes place. Furthermore, those in training are in constant marked caloric excess as they are continually gaining weight. In one study, 60 percent of the wrestlers had diabetic-type glucose tolerance curves, 10 percent were being treated with insulin, and 25 percent had diabetic retinopathy.(22) In comparably aged, non-obese Japanese subjects, the incidence of abnormal glucose tolerance tests were approximately 5 percent, and the rate of diabetes about 1 percent —clearly demonstrating that obesity, as seen in the sumo-wrestlers, predisposes diabetes.(20)

Besides weight, exercise is critical to the prevention and management of diabetes.(7) In addition to lowering blood sugar and keeping weight down, exercise seems to increase sensitivity to insulin and probably contributes to the integrity and longevity of the pancreatic beta (insulin secreting) cells.(7)

ARE THE VASCULAR COMPLICATIONS OF DIABETES PREVENTABLE BY DIET AND EXERCISE?

The answer appears to be yes—at least in adult-onset diabetes. The evidence comes from epidemiologic observations that the microvascular lesions of diabetes are not seen in individuals with normal blood sugar levels anywhere in the world. If these vascular lesions were caused by a genetic defect unrelated to high blood sugar (hyperglycemia), then their occurrence would be expected in some persons with normal blood sugar. Since these lesions appear only in hyperglycemic individuals (the diabetic), it suggests that diet and exercise, by preventing or limiting hyperglycemia, can sever the connection and limit the morbidity and mortality from these microvascular lesions.

Epidemiologic studies also indicate that diet influences the rate of coronary and generalized atherosclerosis seen in diabetics. In North America, diabetic coronary disease appears two to ten times more frequently than in some Asian, African, and Latin American societies.(36, 38, 40, 42) This dissimilarity can not be attributed to genetic or racial differences as coronary disease is several times higher in diabetic U.S. blacks than in diabetic Nigerian blacks. So too, death from cardiovascular complications occurs much less frequently in men and women of Japanese ancestry who live in Japan than in Japanese living in Hawaii.(20) These differences can only be explained by variations in diet and work (exercise) habits.

In a comparison of diabetic men and women of Japanese ancestry, on the Island of Hawaii and in Hiroshima, the caloric intake was roughly equal, but the average daily consumption of fat was twice as high in the Hawaiian Japanese. Furthermore, the fat intake of the Hawaiian Japanese was predominantly saturated fat.

In these two groups of matched ancestry, the number of vascular complications of diabetes causing death, especially heart attack, was twice as great in the Hawaiian Japanese and not different from the Hawaiian white population. These findings indicate that vascular complications in diabetes are influenced by the amount of saturated fat in the diet and the resultant blood cholesterol level. Moreover, death due to ischemic heart disease, even in non-diabetic Hawaiians, is three times greater in Hawaiian Japanese than in Japanese diabetics living in Japan. This suggests that saturated fat intake may be a greater risk factor for heart attack than diabetes itself. It clearly indicates that a reduction in fat intake in subjects with diabetes, may be the most important approach to prevention of ischemic heart disease.

As is true for non-diabetics, the rate of coronary disease in diabetic populations is influenced by blood cholesterol levels.(33, 38, 40, 42) Blood cholesterol is elevated in diets high in saturated fat and, to a lesser extent, hyperglycemia itself seems to produce hypercholesterolemia.(44) It has been clearly shown that serum cholesterol is highest in those diabetics under poor control. Thus, the diabetic diet should limit not only the intake of calories but also saturated fat. Egg yolks, fatty meats, butter, and other whole—milk dairy products are even more harmful to the diabetic than the non-diabetic. Table 4-2 indicates our major dietary sources of cholesterol, saturated fat, and polyunsaturated fat.

Table 4–2
Major Sources of Cholesterol, Saturated Fat, and Polyunsaturated Fat

Cholesterol	Saturated Fat	Polyunsaturated Fat
Egg yolk	Lard	Sunflower seed oil
Offal meats	Suet	Corn oil
Shellfish	Pork, bacon, mutton,	Cottonseed oil
Dairy products	and beef fat or	Peanut oil
	dripping	Soyabean oil
	Butter	Safflower oil
	Hard margarines	Soft margarines
	Hydrogenated vegetable	made from these oils
	oils	All nuts except
	Coconut oil	coconut & cashew
	Hard cheeses and	"Oily" fish, e.g.,
	cream cheese	herring, mackerel
	Cream, dairy products	

THE PURPOSE OF THE DIABETIC DIET

Each diabetic diet must be tailored to the individual. In addition, the needs of the insulin-dependent diabetic vary from those of the non-insulin-dependent, obese, adult-onset diabetic. Tables 4-3 and 4-4 outline some of the major differences.

It is now apparent that, when the total daily calories are controlled, diets high in carbohydrate are well tolerated by diabetics.(41) They should curtail the intake of refined sugar, but generous amounts of starch may be consumed when there is no caloric excess. This means considerable

Table 4-3

Dietary Plan for the Insulin and Non Insulin Dependent Diabetic

Plan	Obese Non Insulin Dependent Diabetic	Non Obese Insulin Dependent Diabetic
1. Decrease no. of calories	Yes	No
2. Protect or improve pancreatic beta-cell function	Yes	No (beta cells usually extinct)
3. Increase frequency & no. of feedings	No	Yes
4. Maintain daily consistency of caloric, carbohydrate, protein, & fat consumption	No (if caloric consumption is low)	Yes
5. Time meals consistently	No	Yes
6. Allow extra food for unusual exercise	No	Yes (or reduce insulin injection)
7. Use food to treat or abort hypoglycemia	No	Yes

flexibility in diet. In general, the diabetic should reduce the saturated fat level (see Table 4-2) in his or her diet to about half the suggested level. This energy source can be replaced with unsaturated vegetable fat or starch.

Food exchange lists are available from the American Diabetics Association, 430 N. Michigan Avenue, Chicago, Ill. 60611. The food exchange system affords the diabetic flexibility in choice of foods, while maintaining consistency of total calories and diet composition. For the insulin-dependent diabetic, acquiring a knowledge of dietetics will allow a flexibility in food choice beyond the standard diabetic exchange lists. For the non insulin-dependent diabetic, exchanged lists are usually not necessary, as long as foods high in refined sugar or saturated fat are eliminated and the total caloric intake is reduced.

While the specific diet your doctor prescribes, in terms of content and calories, will be determined by your size and energy expenditure, certain general principals apply. Eat only the number of meals and amounts of foods listed on your meal plan. Do not skip any meals (this is asking for an insulin reaction). Use no refined sugar, saturated fats, or oils such as olive oil. Take no medicine except that prescribed by your doctor. (This is true for anyone but is

Table 4–4

Nutrients in Normal and Diabetic Diets Expressed as Percent of Total Calories

	Starch	Sugar	Total Carbo-hydrate	Fat	Protein	Alcohol
Normal diet	25–35	20–30	45–50	34–45	12–19	0–10
Traditional diabetic diet	25–30	10–15	35–40	40–45 (2/3 saturated)	16–21	0
Modern diabetic diet	30–45	5–15	45–55	25–35	12–24	0–6

of special importance for the diabetic.) Do not eat specially packaged or dietetic foods unless you consult your doctor first. Table 4-5 lists foods not to be eaten, and Table 4-6 lists foods allowed without restriction.

Is Diet Therapy Feasible?

The answer is definitely yes—if the diabetic understands his diet prescription and food exchanges. This is especially true for the most common type of diabetes, adult—onset disease in the overweight person. Diet therapy, especially in conjunction with an exercise program, will not only control the disease, but also reverse it in many people, as both pancreatic beta-cells' function

Table 4–5

Foods Normally Not to be Eaten

Cake	Cookies	Molasses
Candy	Flavored gelatin	Pie
Canned soups	Gravy & sauces	Prepared fruit punch
Carbonated beverages	Honey	Preserves
(except sugar-free)	Jam	Sorghum
Scalloped foods	Jelly	Sweet pickles
Chewing gum	Marmalade	Syrup
(except sugar-free)		
Condensed milk		

Table 4–6

Foods Allowed Without Restriction

Artificially sweetened gelatin	Dietetic catsup
Bouillon (without fat)	Dill pickles
*Calorie-free dietetic soda pop	Lemon juice
Clear broth (with fat removed)	Lime juice
Coffee (without cream or sugar)	Mustard
Tea (without cream or sugar)	Unflavored gelatin

*No more than 1 or 2 bottles in one day. Some brands of diet soft drinks contain sorbitol, mannitol, or other chemicals similar to sugar. They may be metabolized slowly and add considerable calories to the diet.

and sensitivity to insulin are improved. *It has been esti-mated that half of all diabetics in the United States and other affluent societies could be "cured" by reversal of obesity to optimal body weight, and, thereafter, perma-nent restoration of caloric intake not to exceed caloric expenditure.*(46)

In the lean, insulin-dependent diabetic, diet therapy rarely "cures" the disease, but in conjunction with exer-cise, regulation is improved and vascular complications lessened.

SHOULD THE EXERCISING DIABETIC TAKE VITAMINS?

It has been said that of the 160 million dollars spent annually in this country on vitamin preparations, 140 mil-lion produces nothing but expensive urine! The American Medical Association has reported that, "The use of mul-tivitamin preparations as a form of dietary 'insurance' is a common practice, but it is a poor practice. There is little harm so long as the preparations are not used to excess and the practice is not taken as justification for dietary lunacy."(46) Obviously a vitamin prescription may be needed by people who, through ignorance, poor eating habits, or emotional illness have deficient diets. And they may also be indicated for special periods of nutrient de-mand, such as pregnancy, breast feeding, or prolonged illness. However, in the diabetic, the need for supplemen-tal vitamins is rare, since like the vegetarian, he or she must be diet—conscious.

While supplementary vitamins may help children and adults who have inadequate diets, it should be remem-bered that months of deprivation are required to deplete the body's stores of fat—soluble vitamins. A few days of inadequate intake will not precipitate any health crises—except in the mind. Thus, when taking vitamins, follow the recommendation of the American Medical Association and use them only in specific instances of need. *Remember that specific vitamins in therapeutic amounts should be prescribed only in the presence of vitamin deficiencies or increased requirements.*

SPECIAL SUGGESTIONS FOR THE EXERCISING DIABETIC

One problem that a physical fitness program poses for the diabetic is that, as previously discussed, exercise can increase the rate of insulin absorption, depending upon the site of administration. The exact mechanism for increased insulin absorption is uncertain, but it apparently is related to increased blood flow to the area affected by the exercise. Thus, leg exercise has been shown to increase the absorption rate of insulin injected subcutaneously into the thigh or buttock. Because of this tendency, the diabetic is cautioned to use a non-exercised site for his or her insulin injection. If they do not, the risk of a hypoglycemic reaction is significantly increased. (See Figure 4-1.)

While diabetics can inject insulin subcutaneously anywhere in the body, recent studies indicate that exercise has no effect on the absorption of insulin from the arm or abdominal wall. In fact, in these studies, the disappearance of insulin from the abdominal wall was slightly retarded in the post-exercise period. Therefore, for most exercises that require movement of both the upper and lower body, the abdominal wall is the preferable site for an injection that preceeds vigorous exercise (this usually means the morning injection, if the exercise is to be done during the day). For the runner, it appears that either the arm or abdominal wall is adequate. The arm, thigh, and buttock can be used for the evening insulin injection if a second dose is taken. But if exercise is to be done at night, both the morning and evening insulin injections should be given in the abdominal site. (Figure 4–1, page 91.)

How to Prepare for Vigorous Exercise

In preparing for vigorous exercise, the insulin-dependent diabetic must be aware of certain conditions that significantly lower sugar levels. (For example, the hypoglycemic effect of a thigh injection in an exercising leg.) Also, either extremely hot or cold weather causes the body to work harder and expend more energy (i.e., burn more glucose) to maintain its thermostatic status quo. The same is true of diabetics exercising with virus colds or other infections combined with a fever. In women diabetics, the menstrual period and pregnancy require greater energy and, coupled with exercise, can lower the sugar level. In these situations, the diabetic can make one of two adjustments—decrease insulin or increase caloric intake.

Figure 4–1   Recommended insulin injection sites before ▉▉ and after ▨▨▨ exercise.

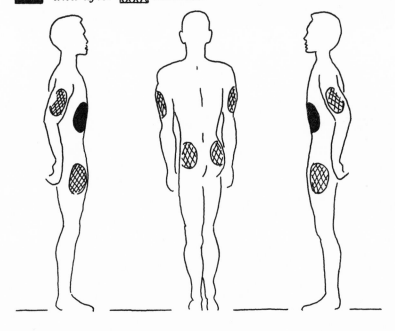

For healthy diabetics exercising under normal circumstances, a reduction of insulin and food intake, except for a small increase of readily usable carbohydrate immediately before exercise, will strike an ideal balance. For the competitive athlete, maximal performance is achieved when insulin is left unchanged and carbohydrate is taken just before the competition. In following this prescription, Bobby Clark a superstar in professional hockey, explains, "I tried to change insulin doses to help with control, but I found it was easier for me to change my food intake to conform with my changing level of activity."(5)

To avoid an insulin reaction during competition, some diabetics try for a slight spill as they commence their exercise. For example, Bill Talbert, the tennis player, states, "I try to be slightly on the plus side and stay there during my exercise."(5) It has been shown that, in response to vigorous exercise, the diabetic has a greater fall in blood glucose than the normal person. Therefore, if the diabetic is to avoid hypoglycemia during exercise, he or she must start it with either a mildly elevated blood sugar level or some rapidly absorbable carbohydrate in their stomach.

However, let me caution that the opposite condition, high blood sugar, will also undermine sports proficiency, not to mention long—term health. While a slight rise in blood sugar before vigorous exercise will improve perfor-

Table 4–7

Recommended Pre-Exercise Diabetic Snacks

Apples	Graham crackers
Bananas	Junior baby foods
Beef jerky	Maple sugar candy
Breakfast squares	Milk
Cheese & crackers	Nuts, especially peanuts
Chocolate-covered wafers	Peanut butter crackers
Cookies	Potato chips
Cupcakes	Raisins
Dried fruit	Sweet rolls
Donuts (plain)	Various sandwiches

mance and prevent an insulin reaction, too much can be dangerous. Table 4-7 lists some acceptable pre-exercise foods that combine short—term (concentrated sugar) energy and long term (slower acting carbohydrates and proteins) energy.

How to Handle an Insulin Reaction While Exercising

For most diabetics, an insulin reaction begins with a light-headed, dizzy sensation, followed by a feeling of weakness, palpitations, and cold, clammy skin. Individual symptoms can vary markedly; for some, personality changes may occur, with a belligerent, ill-tempered demeanor not uncommon. Most diabetics quickly learn to read their own signals of low blood sugar. If exercising when the signals arrive, stop immediately and drink or eat a quick-acting sugar such as honey, orange juice, or a candy bar. It is imperative that you act promptly, as judgment is one of the first things to go during an insulin reaction. The most efficient remedy is sugar already dissolved in fluid; however, sugar usually acts rapidly enough when eaten. No exercising diabetic should ever be without an emergency sugar supply. Life-savers candy are handy and efficient, entering the blood stream even faster than sugar, because they contain corn syrup, a form of glucose. Not recommended are chocolate candy bars—a messy food that acts slower than other candies, because of its relatively high fat content.

How much sugar is enough? That depends on individual physical and activity factors. Guidelines do exist, however, and for most diabetics 10-15 grams of glucose is sufficient to reverse a reaction. The Joslin Clinic, in its Diabetes teaching-guide advises: "Treat all reactions immediately. Take a simple fast-action sugar and allow it 10 to 15 minutes to act. Repeat the same dose of sugar if [there is] no improvement with the first."

Table 4–8

Sugar Content of Recommended Foods for Diabetic Insulin Reactions

Corn syrup (Karo)	1 tbsp	= 15 grams
Cube sugar	2 cubes	= 12 grams
Honey	1 tbsp	= 16 grams
Jam	1 tsp	= 14 grams
Jelly	1 tsp	= 13 grams
Life Savers	3 Candies	= 10 grams
Maple syrup	1 tbsp	= 13 grams
Orange juice	½ cup	= 10 grams
Sugar (1 packet = 1 tsp)	2 packets	= 8 grams
Sweetened soda pop	½ cup	= 20 grams

The amount of sugar that the exercising diabetic carries with him does not have to be a precise dosage. As Dr. O. Charles Olson, Director of the Diabetes Education Center at the Deaconess Hospital in Spokane, Washington, states, "Actually a couple of rolls of Life—savers or half a dozen sugar cubes, in most instances does the trick nicely."(5)

If you have no sugar (something the diabetic—and most importantly, the exercising diabetic—should never be without), then send a companion for some, while you lie down, relaxed and motionless, to expend as little energy as possible. Common sense dictates that the diabetic should never exercise alone, and that his or her companion should be able to treat an insulin reaction. It is tempting to exercise alone, especially when running and jogging. Yet, while diabetics have accomplished incredible feats alone, reason dictates that no sports or conditioning activity should be pursued without a companion.

In summary, the exercising diabetic should take some added carbohydrates just before vigorous, sustained physical effort; must always have sugar nearby; should not pursue his or her activity alone. See Table 4-8 for some common foods suggested for reactions, listed with their sugar content.

Skin Infections and the Exercising Diabetic

One of the fears instilled in many exercising diabetics is that they are highly prone to infection. This has caused almost hysterical concern among some diabetics regarding the consequences of everything from ingrown toenails, superficial cuts and abrasions, to common viral colds. In hopes of avoiding these minor problems, diabetics religously consume daily quantities of vitamins C, B_{12}, E and others. While this certainly leads to expensive urine, it only benefits the diabetic on a balanced diet psychologically. Otherwise, the young and middle-aged diabetic under good control can anticipate healing as rapidly and with no more chance of infection as the non-diabetic.

For the diabetic over 50, healing may be retarded and the chance of infection increased if vascular occlusive disease is present. Here, slow healing is due not to the diabetes, but rather to poor circulation. If circulation is inadequate to meet the metabolic demands of the tissues, then healing will be retarded and the chance of infection increased.

While young diabetics should not worry about healing and infection, common sense dictates that anyone on a rigorous exercise program pay good attention to any cuts, abrasions, or blisters. This is especially true of the feet where the affected area is difficult to keep clean. If you do sustain a foot injury, give it immediate attention by resting, soaking and cleansing the injured area, and controlling the diabetes.

This latter important aspect cannot be too strongly stressed. It is discouraging to hear some authorities state that half of the young diabetics never experience good control. It is the expressed intent of this book to provide a means of reducing that figure to near zero, and preventing the disease in most adults.

Exercise and Some Advantages of Being Diabetic

Some ask if I am joking when I imply there may be advantages to being diabetic. Not at all! Diabetics, of necessity, must acquire self-discipline in relation to their own diet, exercise, and, if required, medicine. This self-discipline carries over into other activities demanding daily determination and stick-to-itiveness, such as sports, school, and work. Mary Tyler Moore has said, "I feel very positive about my 'malfunction.' It means I go to the doctor more than most people and exercise more than most people and watch my diet more than most people. And as a consequence, I think I'm healthier than most people." The controlled, young and middle—aged diabetic is often in better health than his obese, non-exercising, non-diabetic friends. And since the diabetic has regular physical examinations, other physical problems have an excellent chance of being detected earlier than in the non-diabetic, who is likely to have physical check-ups more sporadically.

Since exercise is a vital factor in treating diabetes, the fun of pursuing it can be a major priority in the life of the diabetic. While the non-diabetic may skip a set of tennis because he feels guilty "having fun" instead of finishing work, the diabetic realizes that exercise is vital to his daily medical treatment, and, only by pursuing it, can he be at his best at work. Dan Rowan, the television personality, exercises daily, does body-building calesthenics twice a week, and plays tennis four to six times a week, as part of his other conditioning program. Most people would love to have a doctor *prescribe* recreation like this for them!

Another positive aspect of diabetes is that it, like any chronic disease, tends to make the stricken individual realize he or she has a fixed period of time on this earth and that life will surely go on without us. None of us are indispensible! This realization will hopefully make us more appreciative of our time, and help us to plan our daily activities, both work and play. There are twenty-four hours in the day, and most people require eight hours of sleep. That leaves sixteen hours for work, play, and meditation. Almost none of us uses all those hours wisely, and many of us waste at least four or more hours a day. At that rate, we waste one year every six years. With an age expectancy of 72 years, the average person may be wasting eight years of his life! But for someone who better structures his days, such as the active and well-controlled diabetic, life is active living, all the time.

Up to this point, I have been speaking generally about diabetes and the value of exercise for diabetic prevention and control. Now, in the remainder of the book, we get to the nuts and bolts of *your* exercise program. In these chapters you will not once hear me use the word diabetic —as I make no distinction between the diabetic and non-diabetic. This is for two reasons: First, with the information already given about exercise, insulin, carbohydrate requirements, diet, hypoglycemia, and tips for the exercising diabetic, you are already armed with enough knowledge to pursue any exercise program you desire. You, the overt, chemical, or prediabetic, now know the lifesaving importance of your exercise program. You also realize that diabetic cardiovascular and musculoskeletal systems respond to exercise in a manner identical to non-diabetics.

Second, I make no mention of the diabetic because most diabetics have non-diabetic siblings, spouses, and friends, and exercise programs are as important to the health and vitality of these people as they are to diabetics. Moreover, we are usually more faithful to an exercise program if we do it with others. So I urge you, the diabetic, to encourage your non-diabetic relatives and friends to join you in exercising. Everyone will benefit, as you reduce blood pressure and blood cholesterol, lessen the chance of heart attack, stroke, and vascular disease, and acquire new energy and zest, developing a lean, agile body, and improving your spirit and self-esteem. So without further delay, depending on your age, proceed to Chapter 8 or 9 and carry on.

5

How to Live Painlessly with Your Low Back Problem

It's like a lion at the door;
And when the door begins to crack,
It's like a stick across your back;
And when your back begins to smart,
It's like a penknife in your heart;

Charles Perrault (1628–1703),
author of *Mother Goose Tales*

*A*s a busy neurosurgeon, the most common medical problems I see are not brain tumors, ruptured cerebral aneurysms, strokes, or spinal cord injuries, but spine problems involving, primarily, disorders of the lower back. For me, this is gratifying, for most brain tumors are malignant and incurable, while almost all spine problems are correctable.

At one time or another, almost everyone will experience low back pain. A recent U.S. Public Health Service report indicates that seventy million Americans have experienced at least one severe, incapacitating, prolonged episode of low back pain.(10) Our National Center for Health Statistics states chronic and recurring back ailments form the largest single medical ailment.(10) Today, low back pain represents a major national health problem with over fifteen billion dollars spent annually on the treatment for and compensation of low back—problem sufferers. In industry, compensation for low back problems represents a figure in excess of the cost of all other industrial injuries combined.(1)

Experience in Sports Medicine indicates that low back problems are a very common ailment in the athlete and non-athlete alike. The medical team for the Canadian athletes at the 1976 Olympic Games found low back pain a common problem in their highly trained athletes.(12) Many outstanding Olympic athletes tolerate low back pain as a constant problem, and in some cases the disorder has progressed to the point of neurologic involvement—with the athlete still competing.

What are the causes of low back pain? Why are young, vigorous, physically fit male and female athletes suffering the same symptoms so prevalent in the unfit, sedentary middle-aged? The cause of low back pain is usually mechanical, either a strain of the back muscles or improper postural alignment (with or without weakness of certain muscles). Fortunately, this problem can be successfully treated in most people with the simple back exercises, postural correction program, and helpful hints outlined in this chapter. There is a correct way to sit, walk, stand, and carry out normal activities of daily living so that the low back and pelvis are in the correct postural alignment. Likewise, there is a correct way to lift. Those with low back problems must learn to avoid certain movements and activities which place excessive stress in this area of the body.

A small percentage of people with low back problems will not only have low back pain, but also pain that radiates from the back into the buttock and/or down one or both legs. Coughing, sneezing, straining to pass urine or a bowel movement usually makes the leg pain worse. Numbness may be felt, usually in the foot either over the medial half or along the lateral side. This pattern of pain is called sciatica and suggests a ruptured disc is pressing on a nerve root.

Discs are the fibrocartilagenous cushions between the vertebra. As we age, they lose fluid content, becoming slightly narrower, and cause all of us to shrink slightly in height. The outer more fibrous capsule of the disc, called the *annulus fibrosus,* may also tear, allowing the disc to rupture in the back of the disc space and compress the nerve root as it exits from the spine. Most simple ruptures can be treated successfully with a period of bedrest, muscle relaxants, anti-inflammatory medicines, analgesics and, later, exercises. A minor percentage of sufferers, with neurological deficits, i.e., a reflex absence at knee or ankle, weakness of ankle or great toe extension, or persistent pain and numbness, will require surgical excision of the ruptured disc. The success of such surgery should exceed 90 percent. Following surgery, the patient should adhere to the exercises and advice given in this chapter.

A third and very small group of people with low back problems suffer from mechanical malalignment of the vertebrae——*spondylolisthesis.* This diagnosis is established by x-ray of the back. If there is instability documented by further malalignment, as the back is placed through flexion and extension maneuvers, then a surgical procedure of lumbar fusion may be indicated.

Another small group of people may experience back pain due to an abnormal lateral curvature of the spine called *scoliosis.* In children, severe scoliosis may require surgical correction, which is an extensive and time consuming procedure. For most, however, the scoliosis is mild and can be pain free if the exercises and hints in this chapter are followed. Only a physician, and especially an orthopedist or neurosurgeon, is properly qualified to evaluate and treat your low back problem. Therefore, the exercises and advice in this chapter are directed primarily at the person with low back pain but without neurologic deficit, or the person who has already had concern for a ruptured disc or spinal instability eliminated by appropriate medical consultation.

THE MECHANISM OF LOW BACK STRAIN

The lower back is composed of five mobile, lumbar vertebrae with cartilagenous cushions—or discs—between them, and the fused bones of the sacrum and coccyx, which forms the back of the pelvis. It is in the area of the lumbar vertebra, that all forward (flexion) and backward (extension) movement of the back occurs. Movement is greatest and thus stress is maximal between the sacrum and fifth lumbar vertebra and between the fourth and fifth lumbar vertebra. That is why more than 80 percent of all lumbar disc-ruptures occur at those levels. Because the lumbar spine curves forward, the vertebra are supported by the back muscles, much in the same way as a leaning pole may be supported by guy-wires.

The position of the pelvis, which is controlled by the hip and abdominal muscles, affects the position of the low back. The forward curvature of the low back increases when the upper pelvis rotates forward and downward. The result is a swayback appearance or what medically is termed increased *lumbar lordosis.* This position causes the muscles and ligaments of the back to become shortened and tight. Pain may result without exertion, and almost certainly will appear with any sudden movement or exertion. This condition occurs when there is weakness of the abdominal muscles and the gluteal muscles of the buttocks.

For most, however, it occurs when care is not paid to achieving good posture, the position of one's body during activity and rest. Good posture is achieved by rotating the top of the pelvis backward which flattens the curve in the low back. The section on exercises in this chapter is designed to strengthen the abdominal and gluteal muscles and stretch out tight back muscles. When this is achieved, lordosis is replaced with a flat low back, and the symptoms of strain——namely pain——will vanish.

Ways to Reduce Backstrain Allowing You to Function with Your Low Back Problem Through Correct Posture

Standing and Walking

1. Stand with your low back erect and as flat as possible. By squeezing your buttocks, and sucking in and tensing your abdomen, you straighten your lower back.
2. Bend at the knees when you must lean, as when leaning over a wash basin. Avoid leaning whenever possible and squat with a straight lower back if possible.
3. Avoid high heeled shoes; they shorten your Achilles tendons and increase lumbar lordosis.
4. Avoid standing for long periods of time, but if you must, alternate left foot and right foot, and if possible, the bent knee position (as on a stool).
5. When standing, don't lean back and support your body with your hands. Keep your hands in front of your body and lean forward slightly.
6. When turning to walk from a standing position, move your feet first, and then the body.
7. Open doors widely enough to walk through comfortably.
8. Carefully judge the height of curbs before stepping up or down.

Sitting

1. Sit so that your lower back is flat or slightly rounded outward—never with a forward curve.
2. Sit so that your knees are higher than your hips;this may require a small footstool for a short person in a chair too high.
3. Hard chair backs that begin contact with your back 4 to 6 inches above the seat, and provide a flat support throughout the entire lumbar area, are preferable.
4. Do not sit in soft or overstuffed chairs or sofas.
5. Avoid sitting in swivel chairs or chairs on rollers.
6. Never sit in the same position for prolonged periods—get up and move around.

Driving

1. Push front seat forward so that your knees will be higher than your hips, and the pedals are easily reached without stretching.
2. Sit with back flat, do not lean forward.
3. Add a flat back-rest if your car seat is soft or if you're travelling a long distance.
4. If on a long trip, stop every 30 to 60 minutes, get out of your car and walk for several minutes, tensing buttocks and abdomen to flatten the back.
5. Always fasten seat belt and shoulder harness.
6. Be sure your car seat has a properly adjusted headrest.

Bedrest

1. Sleep or rest only on a flat, firm mattress. If one is not available, place a bedboard of no less than ¾ inch plywood under the mattress. A board of less thickness will sag, preventing proper spine alignment.
2. When sleeping, the preferred position is on your side, both arms in front, and knees slightly drawn up toward your chin.

3. Do not sleep on your stomach.
4. When lying on your back, place a pillow under your knees, as raising the legs flattens the lumbar curve.
5. When lying in bed, don't extend your arms above your head, relax them at your side.
6. If your doctor prescribes absolute bed rest, stay in bed. Raising your body or twisting and turning can strain your back.

Lifting

1. When lifting, let the legs do the work, using the large muscles of the thighs instead of the small muscles of the back.
2. Squat directly in front of the object you plan to lift, bending your knees and going down as far as necessary with the legs, not the back.
3. Do not twist your body, face the object.
4. Never lift with your legs straight.
5. Don't lift heavy objects from car trunks.
6. Don't lift from a bending forward position.
7. Don't reach over furniture to open and close windows.
8. Tuck in the buttocks and pull in the abdomen.
9. Only lift holding the object close to your body.
10. Lift a heavy load no higher than your waist, a light load no higher than the shoulders, as greater height increases lumbar lordosis.
11. To turn while lifting, pivot your feet, turning your whole body at one time.

EXERCISES FOR LOW BACK PAIN

The ten basic low back exercises that are listed in Table 5–1 and illustrated in the Appendix constitute a potent, effective means of eliminating low back pain. They can easily be done in less than fifteen minutes per day and should be performed daily for maximum effectiveness. Unless specifically prescribed by a physician, these exercises should *not* be done by a person with sciatica (pain radiating from the back, out and down the leg). Sciatica involves irritation of one or more nerve roots as they leave the spine. It is usually due to traction or stretching of a nerve root, or pressure on a root from a ruptured disc. Sciatica may be aggravated by these exercises.

Even in the absence of sciatica, the exercises should not be done if severe back pain is experienced at rest. Wait until the back pain is gone before embarking on the exercise program.

The exercises should be carried out on a hard, flat surface with adequate padding. A tumbling mat is ideal, but a thick rug with underpadding is fine. A thick blanket or quilt added to a thin rug, will also suffice. A pillow placed under your neck, for those exercises done lying down, will make you more comfortable. Wear loose clothing or underclothes.

One must be cautious not to overdo in the beginning. The exercises must always be started slowly and carefully, to allow muscles to loosen up gradually. Never use jerking or snapping movements. Relaxing before exercising aids in achieving the maximum benefit from the exercises. Heat treatments before you start can aid in relaxing tight muscles. Do not be alarmed if the exercises produce some mild to moderate discomfort, which may persist for up to a half-hour. If frank pain occurs, and does not vanish quickly with cessation of the exercise, do no more exercises until you have checked with your doctor—preferably a neurosurgeon or orthopedist.

The exercises should be done every day, twice a day in the beginning. If you are unable to exercise most days of the week, it is better not to do them at all than to exercise once or twice a week. Many find that doing them when they first get up in the morning, and again at night just before retiring, are the most convenient times. Others, bored by the exercises, find that doing them while the TV set is on relieves the monotony.

Each person should progress at his or her own pace. Three repetitions of every exercise for the first several days is recommended. Then, one may add a repetition or two daily to each exercise, repetitions that can be done with relative ease and comfort. In this way, gradually build to the minimum desired number of repetitions as later outlined for each exercise.

It can not be stressed too strongly that all exercises must be executed slowly and smoothly. If one or more of the exercises produces significant discomfort, it should be discontinued for several days while the remainder are carried out. An attempt to resume the exercise very slowly, smoothly, and carefully, with fewer repetitions, can then be made several days later. If pain is experienced even then, do not resume that exercise without first checking with your doctor.

A Word of Caution

If one carries out this back exercise program faithfully, he or she can anticipate participating in virtually any

Table 5–1

Exercise		Description
1.	Back Flattener	6, pp. 188–189
2.	Single Knee Raise	13, p. 192
3.	Single Knee Hug	14, p. 192
4.	Double Knee Hug	15, pp. 192–193
5.	Single Leg Raise	16, p. 193
6.	Partial Sit-up	24, pp. 196–197
7a	Advanced Sit-up	25, p. 197
7b	Advanced Mod. Sit-up	26, p. 198
8.	Sitting Bend	27, pp. 198–199
9.	Deep Knee Bend	29, pp. 199–200
10.	Posture Check	8, p. 190

physical activity. When your low back discomfort is relieved for at least one month, I encourage you to progress
to Chapter 8 or 9 depending on your age. A word of caution,
though, about those physical pursuits that can easily produce low back strains and, thus, re-injure your back. Basically, one should avoid rough physical contact, twisting,
sudden impact, or backward arching.

The high risk exercises are: calisthenics involving the
back, such as backward arching movements, toe touches,
hip twists, straight leg sit-ups, or straight leg raises, backward diving movements, football, handball, ice hockey,
sledding—especially on a toboggan—snowmobiling, soc-
cer, squash, tennis, trampoline, volleyball, and weight lifting.

Activities in the moderate risk group include: backpacking, baseball, basketball, bowling, golf, horseback riding,
ice skating, jogging, Ping-Pong, skiing, and softball.

Exercises with minimal risk of back strain include: bicycling, hiking, swimming, and walking.

Still, life must be fun and I am sure most people with
back problems will want to participate in some sports activities once their pain is relieved and they learn to trust
movement rather than fear it. I certainly am not saying
not to do so. I, personally, have suffered from back strain.
Yet, the enjoyment and emotional release derived from
tennis and distance running is, for me, very important,
and I still actively compete year round in both sports. In
my mind, the satisfaction justifies the risk. Thus, I point
out the various activities that are more likely to produce
back injuries so that you are aware of the risk, fully responsible for your decisions, and ready to recognize symptoms connected to the sport you choose.

There are tips that can reduce the risk of back injury for
most of the activities listed above. First, for any sport, always warm up slowly and include some back stretching
exercise. Avoid or use caution with any movement that
arches the back backward, such as spiking a volleyball,

hitting a twist serve or deep overhead in tennis, backward flips on a trampoline, and lifting any heavy weights in the clean and jerk or military press. If you want to use weights, concentrate on many repetitions of a lighter weight for arm curls and bench presses, while avoiding the lifts that cause maximal stress to the low back.

Thus, intelligently pursued, with adequate preparation, you can play a variety of sports potentially hazardous to the low back with little risk of back injury. There is no substitution for the faithful, daily execution of an appropriate back exercise program. It is with you alone that the ultimate responsibility for eliminating back problems and injuries lies.

6

Fitness for the Physically Disabled

Know then thyself, presume not God to scan;
The proper study of mankind is man.

Alexander Pope (1688–1744)

$\mathcal{J}$he physical disabilities covered in this chapter include hereditary (congenital) birth defects, all in—utero birth defects, as well as the acquired loss of one or more limbs, anatomically (by amputation) or functionally (by neurological impairment). While recreation means different things to different people, for most, it provides a pleasurable and purposeful means of using leisure time. For the severely disabled, especially those who cannot work or find employment and, thus, not by choice, may have entire lives of leisure, recreation may assume a far more significant role. For many handicapped people, it will be the one activity that brings them out in the world, integrated in society.

Sports activity, in addition to providing important social

contact, may also provide the opportunity to improve muscular function in a particular disability, thus complementing whatever physiotherapy may have been started. Recreational activities may even accomplish specific functional treatment objectives not attainable with other therapeutic media. Physical motions not possible through various occupational therapy crafts have been witnessed during games. Of uppermost importance is the keen interest and spirit that sports and games generate, increasing motivation, physical tolerance, and self-confidence, when emphasis is taken off the disability and placed on the activity.

Recreational activity may, additionally, provide a sense of freedom otherwise unknown to the disabled. Consider the different perspective an otherwise wheelchair-bound paraplegic has from the saddle of a horse, the seat of a kyack shooting the rapids, or from a sailplane soaring high above the earth. Aside from the physical benefits from exercise, the emotional highs are even greater for the physically handicapped. The aesthetic enjoyment, opportunity for personal expression, and the enriching life experience attained through physical activities is, I believe, even greater for the disabled. The therapeutic benefits are obvious.

HISTORICAL PERSPECTIVES

Man's genuine concern for and systematic efforts to aid the handicapped date back about 200 years. One of the early leaders whose philosophical and educational writings provided spiritual impetus was the Swiss-French philosopher Jean Jacques Rousseau.

For the first one hundred of those 200 years, essentially all the pioneers in work for the handicapped were European. French leaders included Jean Itard, Eduard Sequin, and Alfred Binet, whose research was on the mentally handicapped. Sign language for the deaf was developed by Abbe Sicard and writing for the blind by Louis Braille. Johann Pestalozzi was a leader in Switzerland, Maria Montessori in Rome, and Alfred Adler and Agust Aickhorn in Austria.

In the last half century, the United States has become the leader in many aspects of research, services, and progress for children and adults with physical, mental, and emotional disabilities. The economic resources that provide freedom of investigation in the United States have afforded a climate for unsurpassed growth of theory, research, experimentation, and demonstration projects. Since World War II, especially, there has also been a marked improvement in public attitudes toward the disabled. This has resulted in new legislation, funding, institutions, and many novel approaches toward treatment of the handicapped.

PHYSIOLOGY OF EXERCISE FOR THE DISABLED

It has been shown that the physically handicapped, through exercise, can achieve the same physical and emotional benefits as those of us not disabled. In one study, the fitness test results of a group of wheelchair athletes was compared with those of non-wheelchair athletes. The same increased aerobic capacity and overall training effect was seen for arm work as has been shown for leg work, such as in runners. The wheelchair athletes had significantly higher oxygen uptakes and lower resting and exertional heart rates.(25) Other studies have shown the increased blood flow in regularly exercised arms as compared with those not so physically trained.(38) It is clear that, through equivalent aerobic activity using other portions of the body, the handicapped can reap all the emotional and physical benefits from exercises in this book (listed in Table 1–1, page 34, and discussed in Chapter 1).

SELECTION OF A RECREATIONAL PURSUIT

Able-bodied individuals have varied personalities, temperaments, and physical characteristics that result in different recreational preferences; the presence of physical disability does not change these inherent traits. Although most handicapped people can participate in most recreation pursuits with special equipment, thought should be given to some special considerations. First, it is important that the particular physical activity provide an opportunity for enjoyment and success, while not being potentially dangerous because of the specific disability.

There will be differing needs, experience, and implications of the particular medical affliction: The requirements and approach for the congenital paraplegic from a *myelomeningocele,* the paraplegic from an athletic injury, and the paraplegic from terminal cancer, multiple sclerosis, or some other progressive disease are vastly different. People recovering from an injury or illness must be guided toward activities requiring progressively increased physical strength and endurance, while those afflicted with relentlessly progressive illness should be involved with activities they can pursue regardless of diminishing physical activity.

The choice of an activity, though, must reflect the tastes of the individual too, the type and degree of handicap, and to a large extent especially, his or her determination and motivation. A flexible approach is required for each person, especially when multiple handicaps, coordination problems, and strength deficits complicate the picture. In addition, the variation in duration of the handicaps and natural course of the affliction, must be taken into account.

Money enters the picture also, as many disabled people are not well off financially and some sports are quite expensive. I believe, however, that the disabled should never adopt the attitude that cost will prevent their participation in a sport. Given adequate determination and motivation, financial barriers can be overcome—there are many ways money can be raised for special equipment, courses, and so on.

What makes many of these pursuits possible is special physical equipment. The key to skiing for the amputee, for instance, is the outrigger. This is a ski tip attached by a hinged mount to an adjustable metal crutch. Amputee skiers use two outriggers in a manner similar to using a crutch, except that when skiing they lean forward on the outriggers for balance. Some outriggers are fitted with a spring-loaded spike that plunges several inches into the snow from the center of the ski. This acts much like a conventional ski pole to afford assistance on the level or uphill. With practice and conditioning and the outriggers, amazing performances on even the most difficult slalom courses have been achieved.

The unilateral leg amputee who is otherwise in good condition often finds slalom water skiing quite easy to master. Here, only the standard ski is used and no special equipment is required. A trick that aids in reducing the force on the one leg at the start is to lean forward over the ski before the boat accelerates. Once the boat accelerates, the amputee in this position in essence body-planes to the upright position, then stands on the one leg. The increased surface area of the chest aids in having the ski on top of the water more quickly. Water skiing can also be enjoyed by the blind, as well as arm amputees.

You might wonder how the lower extremity amputee can sky dive and withstand the impact on landing. This does require some planning. The answer can be taken from the space program. Just as our spacecraft parachuted into the ocean, the amputee sky diver can find a soft landing in a lake, reservoir, or similar body of water. As the Russians utilize the desert, so, too, a sandpit can serve as an alternative landing site.

Paraplegics and bilateral lower extremity amputees have taken up a variety of activities, some of which I would be hesitant to try. I can assure you, I have no desire to duplicate the mountain climbing, repelling down sheer mountain cliffs, nor parakiting behind a speeding car—exploits enjoyed by uni- and bilateral leg amputees.

Scuba diving presents no problem when a special shortened "wet suit" with flippers firmly attached to the suit legs just below the stumps is worn. Sailing, sledding, canoeing, angling, rock climbing, cave exploring, hang gliding, and even wheelchair parakiting behind a moving car have been done. Horseback riding can be enjoyed by the bilateral amputee with or without prostheses. A safety belt similar to those used in automobiles can be employed to hold one in the saddle. Riding is also a favorite activity of many suffering from mental illness; cerebral palsy; congenital, hereditary, neurological, and traumatic conditions; the blind, deaf, and limbless. While some may not progress beyond walking on a horse, others will acquire new skills and freedom and be able to join leisure activities on a par with able-bodied riders. Regardless of skill, all experience a feeling of freedom and independence. While riding, they can largely forget their disability and, regardless of the terrain, go where they want. The outdoor feel of sun and wind on the face, the sights, sounds, and smells provide immense enjoyment. Physical benefits besides aerobic exercise include improvement in balance, coordination, body awareness, agility, relaxation, and stretching of tight structures. The element of danger is also present—which most disabled people have lacking in their lives and find immensely stimulating.

Today, riding therapy has assumed a major role in the treatment of children with physical, emotional, and intellectual handicaps. Elsebet Bödtker of Norway, a trained physiotherapist, is a recognized pioneer in this field. Recognizing the unique therapeutic values of horseback riding, both in developing physical skills and in gaining confidence, she started the world's first riding school for disabled children in 1953. Twenty years later in 1973, the school hosted a world conference on riding therapy. Only very recently has the United States acknowledged riding therapy with wide acceptance. However, the Cheff Center for the Handicapped, located in Augusta, Michigan, is the world's largest riding school. This center has also published an enthusiastically accepted, excellent training manual on therapeutic riding for the handicapped.

Another aspect of riding is that disabled riders can participate in riding clubs, especially on the social and organizational side. They can easily assist at horse shows by judging, and in many other ways. Finally, there are carefully graded competitions for the disabled. The Scandinavian countries devised these competitions which have been widely copied.

Water sports have their own special attraction that many disabled people find to be the best outlet for their abilities. Some of those safely pursued by the handicapped include fly, float, and deep sea fishing, canoeing, kayaking, rowing, sculling, sailing, waterskiing, power boating, snorkeling, and scuba diving.

It is unfortunate that the potential benefit to be derived by the disabled from water sports is not more widely recognized. Fishing, which can be as simple or complicated as the angler wishes it to be, can provide a thrilling awareness of the natural environment. It can also easily be enjoyed from a wheelchair or deck chair. A harness or fixed, vise-type pole-holder allows for one-handed fishing. Special light-weight rods, spinning reels, and other devices for the handicapped fisherman are available through catalogues and customer service personnel from several companies including Orvis Co., L. L. Bean, and Abercrombie and Fitch. Sailing and canoeing contain more of a risk element, which most youngsters and some oldsters find very stimulating.

It is the awareness of a new sense of freedom that is perhaps the greatest reward experienced by the disabled who participate in water sports. For those with restricted movement, this involvement is like living in another dimension where the frustrations and difficulties in walking can be forgotten.

Today, in the late twentieth century, we live in an era of super-sophisticated technology. This is certainly not all bad, and for the disabled, definitely beneficial. Certainly one of the most technical, competitive recreations for the handicapped is target shooting for the quadriplegic. Two physicians from the Sheba Medical Center, Tel-Hashomer, Israel, devised a new flexible spring-coil, multi-directional mounting device enabling competitive target shooting for individuals with severe bilateral upper and lower extremity physical handicaps, and even proposed rules based on severity of paraplegia.(36) Figure 6-1 shows a quadriplegic sitting in his wheelchair with the rifle at a comfortable height. With both hands free, the spring allows the quadriplegic to aim the gun in the desired direction. The rifle butt is on the shoulder, and either hand can be used to pull the trigger. This device affords the severely handicapped the opportunity and satisfaction of participating in yet another sport.

Of all the disabled, amputees are perhaps the people for whom the widest range of sports is possible. Indeed, a single, partial, upper limb amputee is little disabled for running, race-walking, speed-skating, throwing the javelin or shot-put, Ping-Pong, and a number of other pursuits (see Table 6-1). As regards lower limb amputees, below-knee amputees are significantly more independent than above-knee amputees and bilateral amputees. (33) (There is essentially no difference between above-knee and bilateral amputees.) Lower limb amputees list fishing and swimming among the most popular recreational activities, while running and walking long distances were at the head of the list as most arduous. As might be anticipated, it's as true for the lower limb amputee as it is true for the able-bodied: as age increases, functional independence decreases.

For paraplegics, the wheelchair becomes their "wheels." Organized competitions in archery, basketball,

Figure 6-1

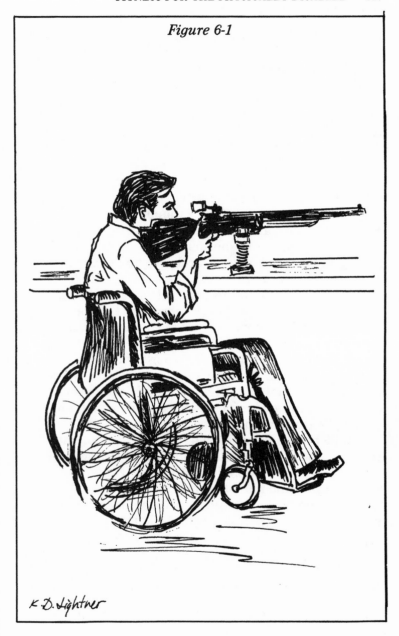

K.D. Lightner

badminton, bowling, croquet, darts, fencing, discus, golf, horseshoes, Ping-Pong, pool, riflery, and road races, including marathons have all been arranged. Other leisure pursuits from square dancing to gardening can be enjoyed from the wheelchair seat. It is recommended that wheelchairs used for outdoor sports have removable arms, swinging or removable footrests, antitrip levers, outer hand rims, and, when desired, pneumatic tires.

For those who become deeply interested in competition, I suggest you contact the International Sports for the Disabled, as meets are regularly held on a regional, national, and international level. The National Wheelchair Games (U.S.) and International Paralympics are held annually with events including shot-put, wheelchair track dashes and relays, weight lifting, archery, table tennis, swimming, and basketball.

The International Sports for the Disabled aims not only to unite national groups in international cooperation, to encourage further development of sports programs, but to provide a forum for the exchange of opinions, experiences, and resources related to sports for the disabled. It also prepares and disseminates international standards, so that individuals are divided into disability classifications to permit fair competition between participants with similar degrees of handicaps.*

Some wheelchair athletes have made their competitive sport the focus of their life. Bob Hall of Belmont, Massachusetts, is a good example. A previous winner of the Boston Marathon and four other marathons in the wheelchair division, Bob began training in November for this year's Boston Marathon (held in April). When the winter cold hit Boston, Bob moved to Florida for his twice-a-day workouts of 8–12 miles. Once a week, usually on Sundays, he went out for a "long run" of 26–29 miles at a 6:20–7:00 minute per mile pace. Midweek, Bob usually also had a "mini-long

---

Official Rule Book and Guide, National Wheelchair Athletic Association.

run" of 18–20 miles. His weekly mileage was around 135 miles with a high of 185.

Since Florida is primarily flat, Bob went to Bermuda for hill work and wind training. He also included a form of weight training with short (30 minute), high-intensity Nautilus weight training workouts two or three times a week.

With such ability and commitment to training, one might think Bob would be unbeatable. But as good as he is, he didn't win this year; a 30-year-old midwesterner from Akron, Ohio, Ken Archer, won the event in 2:38.59, one minute ahead of George Murray of Tampa, Florida. When the ice and cold came to Ohio, Ken Archer took his training indoors, using a treadmill for his daily workouts. Without the beauty, wind, and hills of Bermuda or the warmth of Florida, Archer's faithful adherence to his conditioning routine in which "I kept pushing myself with the use of a treadmill machine," resulted in his victory.

Ironically, it was Bob Hall who sparked Archer's interest in wheelchair marathons. Ken Archer lost his left leg at 21, when it was pinned and crushed between two cars, necessitating amputation. Ken says, of wheelchair marathoning, "I do it because it gives me personal satisfaction."

HOW TO ARRANGE YOUR OWN EXERCISE PROGRAM

The basic requirements of an exercise program for the disabled is the same as that described for the nondisabled. Each exercise program should have three parts: a warm-up, an endurance phase, and a cooling-off period.

The *warm-up* phase should be at least five minutes, and include rhythmic, slow stretching movements of the trunk and limb muscles. This increases blood flow and stretches the postural muscles, preparing the body for sustained activity. To ignore the warm-up is to risk muscle-pulls or more severe injuries. Table A-1 in the Appendix lists fourteen warm-up exercises, and you may choose any combination for your five-minute warm-up period. Vary the exercises on different days to avoid monotony.

The *endurance* phase should last at least thirty minutes. During this period, your cardiovascular system is stressed to increase aerobic capacity. To achieve maximal cardiovascular improvement, exercise vigorously enough during the endurance phase to be breathing deeply, but not falling into greater oxygen debt (grasping for air). As your aerobic capacity increases, you may wish to increase the time and intensity of the endurance phase.

The *cooling-off* phase is too often omitted in exercise. While the endurance phase significantly raises body temperature, increases the heart rate and blood pressure, and

Table 6-1

Recreational Pursuits Especially Appropriate
for the Upper Limb Disabled

Backpacking	Platform tennis
Badminton	Riding
* Bicycling	Rodeo
Bowling	* Roller skating
* Cross-country running	* Running
Darts	Snowshoeing
Fencing	* Soccer
* Ice hockey	* Squash
* Ice skating	Tennis
* Jogging	* Track
* Jumping	* Trampoline
Karate	Tumbling
Lawn bowling	Walking
Ping-Pong	

*Sports for which 30 minutes of continuous activity is sufficient.

builds up lactic acid and other waste products in your muscles, the cooling-off phase allows the bodily functions to return to normal gradually. This helps to eliminate waste products from your muscles, minimizing the chance of stiffness and soreness the next day. The cooling-off phase should last at least five minutes and can be longer if desired. It should include gross body movements that emphasize range of motion of the joints (calisthenics are ideal for this final step in your day's exercise program). It is recommended that you select three exercises and do them for five minutes. To avoid monotony, you may wish to use different exercises from Table A-3 on different days.

For the main endurance phase, I have prepared three tables that list recreational pursuits that are easily adapt-

Table 6–2

*Recreational Pursuits Especially Appropriate
for the Lower Limb Disabled*

Archery (W)	*Kayaking
*Badminton (W)	Lawn bowling (W)
Baseball (W)	Motocross
*Basketball (W)	Motorcycling
Boating	Ping-Pong (W)
Body building (W)	Pool (W)
Bowling (W)	*Rowing
*Canoeing	Sailplanes
Folk dancing (W)	Show jumping
Football (touch or flag) (W)	Softball (W)
Gliding	*Sculling
Golf	Tobogganing
*Handball (W)	*Volleyball (W)
	Weight lifting (W)

(W) demotes use of wheelchair.
*Sports for which 30 minutes of continuous activity is sufficient.

able to the upper limb disabled (Table 6–1), lower limb disabled (Table 6–2), and upper and lower limb disabled (Table 6–3). Those sports for which 30 minutes of continuous activity is sufficient are marked with an asterisk, while those less strenuous, requiring an hour or more, are not. It must be realized, though, that these tables are neither complete nor exclusive. Given burning motivation and desire, with ingenuity, there is virtually no leisure or recreational activity that cannot be mastered——from scuba to sky-diving.

Some of the many athletic organizations for the disabled are presented, as well as a selected bibliography at the end of the book. I encourage you not only to arrange your own exercise program, but to use these resource lists fully.

Table 6–3

Recreational Pursuits Enjoyed by Upper and Lower Limb Disabled

Alpine skiing	Hunting
* Body surfing	Ice fishing
Bowling	Isometrics
Calisthenics	Ping-Pong
Camping	Rock climbing
* Cross-country skiing	Sailing
Dancing	Scuba diving
Darts	Skin diving
Diving (platform)	Sky diving
Fishing	Snorkeling
Gardening	Sports car rallying
Gymnastics	* Swimming
Hiking	Target shooting
Horseback riding	* Waterskiing

*Sports for which 30 minutes of continuous activity is sufficient.

ATHLETIC ORGANIZATIONS FOR THE DISABLED

Blind

1. American Blind Bowling Association
   150 N. Bellaire Ave.
   Louisville, Ky. 40206
   Phone: (502) 896-8039
   James Murrell, Sec.-Treas.

   Founded: 1951. *Members:* 2600. *Regional Groups:* 3;
   Local Groups: 130. Legally blind men and women, 18
   years of age and older, competing in organized tenpin
   bowling. Promotes bowling as a recreational activity
   for adult blind persons; sponsors member leagues;
   runs a yearly mail-o-graphic; sponsors annual cham-
   pionship blind bowling tournament. Presents awards.
   Publications: The Blind Bowler, 3/year. *Convention/-
   Meeting:* annual tournament, May 1979. Cleveland,
   Ohio; 1980 Cincinnati, Ohio.

2. Blind Outdoor Leisure Development
   533 E. Main St.
   Aspen, Colo. 81611
   Phone: (303) 925–8922
   Richard C. Fenton, Exec. Dir.

   Founded: 1969. *Members:* 20. Operates on the "can-do"
   theory for blind people. Aids in the establishment of
   local clubs in order to enable the blind to experience
   the out-of-doors, by skiing, skating, hiking, fishing,
   horseback riding, golf, swimming, camping, and bik-
   ing. Designs and conducts training courses for activity
   leaders; has designed distinctive jackets and bibs to
   identify participants as blind; provides insurance program for participants. Local clubs solicit reduced costs
   for, or free use of sports equipment and facilities.

Deaf

1. **American Athletic Association For The Deaf**
    3916 Lantern Drive
    Silver Spring, Md. 20902
    Phone: (301) 942–4042
    Richard Caswell, Sec.-Treas.

    Founded: 1945. *Members:* 13,500. *Regional Groups:* 7.
    Local Groups: 155. Fosters athletic competition among
    the deaf and regulates uniform rules governing such
    competition; provides adequate competition for those
    members who are primarily interested in interclub
    athletics; provides a social outlet for deaf members
    and their friends. Sanctions and promotes state, re-
    gional, and national basketball tournaments, softball
    tournaments, participation in activities of the Comite
    International des Sports Silencieux and in World
    Games for the Deaf. Maintains AAAD Hall of Fame
    and gives annual Athlete of the Year Award. *Publica-
    tions:* Bulletin, quarterly. *Convention/Meeting:* semi-
    annual—April and September. 1979 Houston, Texas,
    and Cleveland, Ohio; 1980, San Diego, Calif., and India-
    napolis, Ind.; 1981, Buffalo, N.Y., and Hartford, Conn.;
    1982 Miami, Fla., and Vancouver, B.C., Canada.

2. **International Committee of the Silent Sports**
    Gallaudet College
    Washington, D.C. 20002
    Phone: (202) 447–0841
    Jerald M. Jordan, Exec. Sec.

    Founded: 1924. *Members:* 43. Membership composed
    of athletic organizations for the deaf in each of 43
    countries. Provides an international sports competi-
    tion for the deaf, patterned after the International
    Olympic Games. Seeks to promote and develop physi-
    cal education in general, and the practice of sports in

particular, among the deaf; encourages friendly relations between countries with programs in silent sports, and formation of silent sports programs in countries not yet participating. Holds Summer World Games and Winter Games alternately at two-year intervals. All competitors must have severe hearing loss. Awards gold, silver, and bronze medals to first, second, and third place winners of each event. Medals recognizing valuable personal contribution to the Committee are also awarded. The Committee is recognized by the International Olympic Committee. *Publications:* (1) *Bulletin,* quarterly; (2) *Handbook,* irregular. *Convention/Meeting:* biennial congress, held concurrently with Games.

3. United States Deaf Skiers Association
   159 Davis Ave.
   Hackensack, N.J. 07601
   Dan Fields, Pres.

Founded: 1968. *Members:* 310. Promotes skiing, both recreational and competitive, among the deaf and hearing—impaired in the United States. Provides deaf skiers benefits, activities, and opportunities which will further increase their enjoyment of the sport. Encourages ski racing among the deaf and sponsors national and regional races for deaf skiers. Assists in any way possible the selection, organization and training of the United States Deaf Ski Teams for international competition, such as hockey, the World Winter Games for the Deaf. Presents awards. *Committees:* Ice Figure skating; Speed Skating. *Publications:* Newsletter, 4 per year. *Affiliated with:* United States Ski Association. *Convention/Meeting:* biennial—1980 February, Steamboat Springs, Colo.; 1982 Big Sky, Mont.

Paralysis or Limbs Amputation

1. National Foundation For Happy Horsemanship For
   The Handicapped
   Box 462
   Malvern, Pa. 19355
   Phone: (215) 644–7414
   Maudie Hunter-Warfel, Natl. Advisor

   Founded: 1967. Individuals who assist handicapped
   persons in their involvement with horses as a form of
   therapy and rehabilitation. Purpose is to encourage
   and unify the teaching or driving horses to the disabled through the training of personnel, and the ar-
   ranging of exchanges among those who have
   experience in the field. Provides horses and donates
   facilities for their care. Provides films and conducts
   how-to clinics for volunteers. Maintains 200 volume
   library. *Councils:* National Advisory. *Publications:*
   Newsletter, annual. *Convention/Meeting:* biennial:
   1979 September, England.

2. National Handicapped Sports And Recreation Association
   4105 E. Florida Ave., Third Fl.
   Denver, Colo. 80222
   Fred T. Nichol, Pres.

   Founded: 1972. *Members:* 2207. *Local Groups:* 13. Amputees and other handicapped persons who are interested in participating in all kinds of sports. Provides
   veterans and other inconvenienced (handicapped)
   persons an opportunity to experience sports and par-
   ticipatory recreation activities. Sponsors ski clinics
   and publishes an amputee ski technique manual. *Publications:* Bulletin, semiannual; also publishes Amputee Ski Technique Manual and Blind Ski Teaching
   Manual. *Formerly:* (1972) National Amputee Skiers

Association; (1977) National Inconvenienced Sportsmen's Association. *Convention/Meeting:* annual.

3. National Wheelchair Athletic Association (Handicapped) (NWAA)
40–24 62nd St.
Woodside, N.Y. 11377
Phone: (212) 424-2929
Benjamin H. Lipton, Chm.

Founded: 1958. Members: 1600. *Regional Groups:* 13. Men and women athletes with significant permanent neuromuscularskeletal disability (spinal cord disorder, poliomyelitis, amputation) who compete in various amateur sports events in wheelchairs. The Association is administered by, and under the jurisdiction of the National Wheelchair Athletic Committee. Members compete in regional events and in the annual National Wheelchair Games, which include competitions in track and field (including pentathalon), swimming, archery, table tennis, slalom, and weightlifting. Qualifying rounds are held in each region to select competitors for the national competition. Selection is made at the completion of the nationals to represent the U.S. team in international competition. Travel expenses for the U.S. competitors are subsidized by the U.S. Wheelchair Sports Fund. Publishes Newsletter quarterly.

4. National Wheelchair Basketball Association
110 Seaton Bldg.
University of Kentucky
Lexington, Ky. 40506
Phone: (606) 257-1623
Stan Labanowich, Ph.D., Commissioner

Founded: 1958. *Members:* 130. Conferences: 24. Wheelchair basketball teams made up of individuals with severe permanent physical disabilities of the lower extremeties. Seeks to provide opportunities on a national basis for the physically disabled to participate in the sport of wheelchair basketball, with its adjunct psychological, social, and emotional benefits, and to maintain a high level of competition through continuing refinement and standardization of playing rules and officiating. Sponsors competitions, maintains hall of fame, compiles statistics, participates in charitable activities. Awards trophy annually to winner of National Wheelchair Basketball Tournament. *Publications:* (1) Weekly Standings and Statistics (November—April); (2) Newsletter, bi-weekly (November—April); (3) Casebook, annual; (4) Directory, annual; (5) National Wheelchair Basketball Tournament Program, annual; (6) Rules Book, annual. *Convention/Meeting:* annual sectional and regional tournaments leading up to the national tournament.

5. North American Riding For The Handicapped Association
C/O Leonard Warner
P.O. Box 100
Ashburn, Va. 22011
Phone: (703) 777-3540
Leonard Warner, Sec.-Treas.

Founded: 1968. *Members:* 200. Individuals and centers for the handicapped. Seeks to promote therapeutic riding for the handicapped, with safety and proper care; to provide appropriate training and certification for instructors working with the handicapped. Makes periodic inspections of riding centers in operation. Provides consultants as lecturers and demonstrators. *Publications:* Newsletter, annual.

6. Special Olympics
1701 K St., N.W., Suite 203
Washington, D.C. 20006
Phone: (202) 331-1346
Eunice Kennedy Shriver, Pres.

Founded: 1968. *Members:* 1,000,000. *Local Groups:* 14,-
000. *Regional Groups:* 8. *State Groups:* 52. Created and
sponsored by the Joseph P. Kennedy, Jr. Foundation to
promote physical education and athletics for the retarded. Local, area and chapter games are conducted
in 50 states, District of Colombia, Puerto Rico and 24
foreign countries. International Special Olympics are
staged quadrennially (next: 1979). Participants range
in age from eight years to adult, and compete in track
and field, swimming, gymnastics, bowling, ice skating,
basketball and other sports. Information materials are
available on organization of programs and participation of athletes. Presents annual awards for service to
program through sports. Maintains speakers bureau;
compiles statistics; sponsors research programs. *Councils:* National Advisory. *Publications:* (1) Newsletter
(restricted circulation), quarterly; (2) List of Chapter
and National Directors, annual; also publishes bro-
chure, guide, instructional manual, and list of state
programs. *Convention/Meeting:* annual conference of
chapter and national directors. 1979 Aug. 9–12, Brock-
port, N.Y.

7. American Coalition of Citizens with Disabilities
    1346 Connecticut Ave., N.W.
    Washington, D.C. 20036
    Phone: (202) 785–4265

BIBLIOGRAPHY OF RECREATIONAL ACTIVITIES FOR
THE HANDICAPPED

Archery
1. Heath, E.G.: *A History of Target Archery,* David and
    Charles, Newton Abbott, Devonshire, Eng., 1973.

Camping
2. Bauman, M. K., Strausse, S.: "A comparison of blind children

from day and residential schools in a camp setting." *International Journal of Education for the Blind,* 11:74–77, 1962.

3. Croucher, N.: *Here to Stay: Disabled people in outdoor centres,* Sports Council, 1978.

4. *Day Camping for the Cerebral Palsied:* New York, United Cerebral Palsy Associations, Inc., *Program Bulletin 11.*

5. Frampten, M. E., Mitchell, P. C.: *Camping for Blind Youth,* New York, American Institute for the Education of the Blind, 1949.

6. Ginglend, D., Gould, K.: *Day Camping for the Mentally Retarded,* New York, National Association for Retarded Children, 1962.

7. Howett, H. H. (ed.): *Camping for Crippled Children,* National Society for Crippled Children and Adults. Chicago, 1945.

8. Kapurch, J. A.: "Camping Through Handicapped." *Am. J. Nurs.,* 66:1794–1797, 1966.

9. Meyers, T.: *Camping for Emotionally Disturbed Boys,* Bloomington, Indiana University, Dept. of Recreation, School of Health, Physical Ed. and Rec., 1961.

10. Schoenbohm, W. F.: *Planning and Operating Facilities for Crippled Children,* Springfield, Ill., Charles C. Thomas, Publishers, 1962.

11. "Summer camps for deaf children" *Alexander Graham Bell Association for the Deaf,* Volta Rev 64:192–199, 1962.

12. Switzer, R. M., Clark M.: "Camping for severely disabled children." *Interclinic Information Bulletin,* 1964.

13. Weller, M. F.: "Camping for handicapped girls, Girl Scout Leader." Girl Scouts of America, New York.

14. Yoffa, G., Lloyd, E. D.: "Camping together." *Cerebral Palsy Journal.*

Gardening

15. Chaplin, M.: *Gardening for the Physically Handicapped and Elderly,* Hippocrene Books, Batsford, 1978.

16. Wilshire, E.R.: "Equipment for the disabled." *Leisure and Gardening,* 2 Foredown Drive, Portsdale, Brighton BN4 2BB.

General

17. *Adapted Sports, Games, Square Dances and Special Events,* Connecticut Society for Crippled Children and Adults, Hartford, Conn.

18. *Adapted Sports in Veterans Administration, Special Services Information Bulletin 1B 6–252.* Washington, D.C., Recreation Service, V.A.

19. Barnett, M. W.: "Blind girl in the troop." *Girl Scout Leader.* April, 1966, pp.20–24.

20. Barnett, M. W.: *Handicapped Girls and Girl Scouting,* A Guide for leaders. New York, Girl Scouts of the United States of America, 1968.

21. Becker, E. F.: *Female Sexuality Following Spinal Cord Injury,* Bloomington, Ill., Accent Spinal Pub., Chever Pub. Inc., P.O. Box 700, 61701.

22. Buell, C. E.: "Developments in physical education for blind children." *New Outlook Blind,* 58:202–206, 1964.

23. Buell, C. E.: *Physical Education for Blind Children.* Springfield, Ill., Charles C. Thomas, 1966.

24. Davies, E. M.: "Let's get moving: Group activation of elderly people." *Age Concern,* 60 Pitcain Road, Mitcham, Surrey, England, 1975.

25. Dendy, E. "Recreation for disabled people - what do we mean." *Physiotherapy,* 64:290–291, 1978.

26. Emes, C.:"Physical Work Capacity of Wheelchair Athletes." *The Research Quarterly of the American Association Health and Physical Education,* 48:209–212, 1977.

27. Fait, H. F.: *Adapted Physical Education,* Philadelphia, W. B. Saunders Co., 1960.

28. Glazier, R. (ed.): *The College Guide for Students with Disabilities,* Cambridge, Mass., Abt. Books, 1976.

29. Guttman, L.: *Textbook of Sport for the Disabled,* HM&M Publishers, Aylesbury 1976.

30. *Holidays for the Physically Handicapped.* Royal Association for Disability and Rehabilitation Annual 1978 edition.

31. Howe, G. T.: "Canoe course for the blind." *Recreation,* 55:131–133, 1962.

32. Juul, K. D.: "European approaches and innovations in serving the handicapped." *Exceptional Child,* 44:322–330, 1978.

33. Kegel, B., Carpenter, M. L., Burgess, E. M.: "Functional capabilities of lower extremity amputees." *Archives Physiology Medicine and Rehabilitation,* 59:109–120, 1978.

34. Kirchman, M. M.: "Rifle Holder." *American Journal of Occupational Therapy,* 19:28, 1965.

35. Obe, N. C.: "Outdoor activities." *Physiotherapy,* 64:294–295, 1978.

36. Ohry, A., Talmor, E. A new flexible spring-coil, multi-directional mounting devise (with proposal of rules) for target shooting by the disabled. *Paraplegia Life* 16:5–7, 1978.

37. *Paraplegia Life.* Published by National Spinal Cord Injury Foundation, 369 Elliot St., Newton Upper Falls, MA 02164.

38. Rathbone, J. L., Lucus, C. *Recreation in Total Rehabilitation,* Springfield, Ill., Charles C. Thomas, 1959.

39. "Recreation for disabled people." *Physiotherapy,* 64:299–301, 1978.

40. *Sports and Spokes,* 4330 East-West Highway, Suite 300, Washington, D.C. 20014.

41. Stewart, F.: *Recreation for the Retarded: a handbook for leaders,* Nat. Soc. of Mentally Handicapped Children, Pembridge Hall, Pembridge Square, London W2 4EP, 1975.

42. Swannell, A. J.: "Medical considerations." *Physiotherapy,* 64:292–293, 1978.

43. Taggie, J. M., Manley, M. S.: *A Handbook on Sexuality After Spinal Cord Injury,* Family Service Dept., Craig Hosp., 3425 S. Clarkson St., Englewood, CO 80110.

44. *Travelability: A guide for Physically Disabled Travelers in the United States,* New York, MacMillan Publishing Co. Inc., 1978.

45. Wakim, K. G., Elkins, E., Worden, R., Polley, H.: "The effects of therapeutic exercise on peripheral circulation of normal and paraplegic individuals." *Archives Physiology Medicine and Rehabilitation,* 30: 86–95, 1949.

46. Weller, M. F.: "Scouting for handicapped girls." *Girl Scout Leader,* May, 1963.

47. Walker, G. M.: "Riding for the Disabled." *Physiotherapy,* 64:297, 1978.

Swimming

48. Mooney, H. V.: "Fabricating of fin prostheses for bilateral amputee." *Orthopedic Prostheses Applied Journal,* September, 221–222, 1966.

49. Register of swimming clubs and organized swimming sessions for the handicapped people. National Association of Swimming Clubs for the Handicapped. 1977–78.

50. Reid, M. J.: "Handling the disabled child in water." *Assoc. of Ped. chartered physiotherapists,* (APCP), Publications 25 Goffs Park Road, Southgate, Crowley West Sussex RH 11 8 AX, England, 1976.

51. Sterling, B.: *Aquatics for the Handicapped,* New York, Hoffman Harris, 1958.

52. "Swimming for the Cerebral Palsied." *Program Bulletin 10,* New York, United Cerebral Palsy Associations, Inc.

53. "Swimming for the Handicapped" *Instructors manual, American National Red Cross,* Washington, D.C.

Other Water Sports

54. *Guide to Fishing Facilities for Disabled Anglers.* National Anglers Council, 5 Cowgate, Peterborough, PEI ILR, 1978.

55. Roberto, K.: "Water Sports." *Physiotherapy,* 64:296, 1978.

56. "State of the Art." *National Recreational Boating for the Physically Handicapped,* Human Resource Center, Albertson, Long Island, NY 11507.

57. *Water Sports for the Disabled,* The Sports Council Advisory Panel, Royal Yachting Association, Victoria Way, Woking, Surrey GU 21 IEQ, 1977.

7

Exercise for the
Post-Heart Attack Patient

Concerning the mode of treatment by which the body and mind are to be preserved ... moderate exercise reduces to order, according to their affinities, the particles and affections which are wandering about the body

> Plato's *Dialogues:* Timaeus speaking to Socrates

NEW CONCEPTS IN TREATING THE HEART ATTACK PATIENT

During the past ten years, dramatic changes have taken place in the in-hospital care of heart attack patients. While out-patient rehabilitation is properly the subject of discussion here, these current concepts of in-patient coronary treatment deserve brief mention.

Most modern hospitals now have coronary care units where the suspected and diagnosed heart attack patients are initially treated. With continuous monitoring, readily available resuscitative equipment, and specially trained personnel, about 50,000 lives a year, which previously would have been lost following a heart attack, are now being saved.

Early ambulation following a heart attack is now routine. Formerly, weeks of bedrest were customary treatment, which heightened the risk of pulmonary embolism and the incidence of profound anxiety and depression; now, the patient is ambulatory within the first three days of an uncomplicated heart attack. Early ambulation also protects against the deconditioning effect bedreast has on the body, and it has significantly reduced the number of people who become invalids after a heart attack.

Hospitals now try to begin a rehabilitation program while the patient is still in the hospital. As a result, the length of hospital stay has been significantly shortened, saving money and space, improving the spirits of the patients, and hastening their return to home and work. The value of early rehabilitation is emphasized by doctors Hackett and Cassen, who write in *Exercise Testing and Exercise Training in Coronary Heart Disease,* that, "Exercise is still the most potent antidote and prophylaxis against depression that we know. There is little doubt that depression heightens mortality. Exercise, therefore, is right on!"(23) It is now estimated that between 80–90 percent of first heart attack patients under 65 years of age will return to work within two to four months.

For those who are hospitalized, post–heart attack rehabilitation is under the direct care of a physician, the rehabilitation is guided and monitored by health professionals. Once patients leave the hospital, however, they are likely to see their doctor only periodically. At home, although armed with advice, they are largely on their own. It is at this phase of recovery that I make an urgent plea to all recovering coronary patients to enroll in a cardiac rehabilitation conditioning program under a doctor's supervision. It is my belief that, with a professionally supervised exercise program, many heart attack victims may not just return to work, but they may restore their hearts to a state far better than before the heart attack and so prevent subsequent attacks. Such a conditioning program will require the elimination or better control of the correctable risk factors for heart desease: hypertension, obesity, diabetes, cigarette smoking and physical inactivity.

WHY CIGARETTE SMOKING IS PREMEDITATED SUICIDE FOR THE HEART ATTACK PATIENT

The avoidance of cigarette smoking deserves special emphasis. A heart attack occurs mainly by one of two mechanisms. There may be an occulsion (blockage) of one or more blood vessels supplying the heart muscle, with resultant *ischemia* (lack of blood supply) that renders the muscle incapable of functioning normally. A second mechanism seen not uncommonly in relatively young, previously asymptomatic individuals, is the development of an arrthymia. In this instance, the sequential filling and emptying of the heart's chambers is disturbed and the net effect is a failure to pump the body's blood. Often, there will be little or no damage to the heart muscle itself. This type of heart attack occurs suddenly, and unless the victim receives immediate cardiopulmonary resuscitation (CPR), the outcome is fatal; the brain cannot survive more than four or five minutes without blood flow. Of the nearly 50 percent of fatal heart attack victims who are dead on arrival at a hospital, most have died of arrythmia, rather than from a massive coronary occlusion.

Smoking Provokes Cardiac Arrythmias

Cigarette smoking causes the more lethal cardiac arrythmia heart attack. In the experience of the Toronto Rehabilitation Centre for post–heart attack patients, almost all the fatal heart attacks were in patients who had refused to stop heavy cigarette smoking.(15) The message is thus clear for the heart attack victim, to repeat, *Smoking Cigarettes Is Suicide!*

Just as oil and water don't mix, neither do exercise and smoking. Cigarette smoke contains carbon monoxide, which competes with oxygen for the same binding site on the red blood cells. To the extent that these bindings sites become occupied with carbon monixide, that much less oxygen can be absorbed and delivered to the tissues. The crucial benefit of exercise, increased aerobic capacity is eroded, because the oxygen transport mechanism is reduced. If you have poisoned your red cells so they can't carry their full load of oxygen, it matters little that your heart has become more efficient at pumping blood or that your muscles extract oxygen more efficiently from your blood. If you smoke, your blood is oxygen-starved.

A final point regarding smoking is an expecially sensitive one to me personally. For the many who wage and win the battle of cigarette smoking, much good can be undone if you are forced to inhale other people's cigarette, pipe, or cigar smoke. Carbon monoxide is the same whether you inhale it from your own or someone else's cigarette. Nonsmokers who subject themselves to smokey night clubs, restaurants, or other enclosed areas will inevitably increase their blood carbon monoxide levels. It is not enough to stop smoking yourself, you must also, whenever possible, avoid others' smoking.

CAN ALL HEART ATTACK VICTIMS EXERCISE SAFELY?

While the vast majority of heart attack patients can safely pursue an endurance exercise program, *it is by no means safe for all.* Some absolute contraindications include: (1) heart muscle damage to a degree that an aneurysm or weakness develops in the heart muscle wall, causing bulging with each heart beat; (2) a recent heart attack; vigorous exercise in the first six weeks after a heart attack can actually predispose to a heart aneurysm; (3) acute heart failure; exercise only aggravates this condition; (4) a progressive or suddenly more severe chest pain (angina) with physical exertion; (5) inflammation of the heart causing myocarditis; (6) grossly irregular heart beats, "multi-focal ectopic arrythmias" with exertions; (7) certain types of congenital and valvular heart disease; (8) recent pulmonary embolism or thrombophlebitis; (9) complete heart block, a condition in which the electrical conduction from the atria to the ventricles is non-functioning, so the chambers beat independently. Additional contraindications include severe anemia, uncontrolled diabetes or hypertension, rare types of epilepsy, recent tuberculosis or recurrent spontaneous pneumothorax, certain types of degenerative arthritis, and chronic low back derangements. *You must be completely clear about your Doctor's diagnosis.*

For those heart patients with absolute contraindications, endurance training must be deferred until these more immediate, life-threatening situations are corrected. Once their condition has stabilized, however, they may also realize the advantage of an exercise program, which include: a slowing of the heart beat and lengthening of the time blood is supplied to the heart muscle, reduction in blood pressure, increased heart output with each beat, increased efficiency of oxygen extraction from the blood by the muscles, mild reduction in clotting time, and decrease in blood triglycerides and cholesterol.

EXERCISE-STRESS TESTING FOR THE HEART ATTACK PATIENT

One of the most significant advancements in coronary treatment during the past few years, has been the extensive use of exercise stress testing not only to determine the appropriate, safe exercise prescription, but also the subsequent upgrading of the prescription. Whereas five years ago, less than 15 percent of American physicians used formal exercise testing to evaluate cardiovascular function, today it is routine.(23) This test is not used to diagnose cardiovascular disease, which is done by a history, cardiac exam, and routine electrocardiogram. Rather, the stress or exercise electrocardiogram is used to evaluate the severity of the heart disease, expose unexpected responses to exertion, as well as to provide a baseline by which the effects of rehabilitation, efficacy of drugs, and varying dosages of drugs can be physiologically assessed.

Exercise testing involves aerobic exertion, preceded by a warm-up and followed by a cooling-off period. It involves only ambulatory patients adequately informed of the methods, risks, and benefits. Carried out under direct medical supervision, with continuous electrocardiogram, heart rate, and blood pressure monitoring, the test has specific criteria for its termination well short of precipitating cardiac arrythmias, myocardial ischemia, exertional hypertension, myocardial infarction, and cardiac arrest.

There are basically three types of exercise tests. The first type which was developed by Master, involves stepping up and down a stair step. This exertion reveals the direct relationship that exists with heart rate, work load, cardiac output, and oxygen uptake until maximum oxygen uptake (VO_2 max.) is reached. Master discovered, by using the electrocardiogram during the step test, that evidence of heart ischemia not detectable in some people at rest could be demonstrated in exertion periods. The electrocardiogram is actually monitored before, during, and after the stepping-exertion phase. Changes in the electrocardiogram, especially a portion called the ST segment that tends to become depressed with cardiac ischemia, are closely observed, as are heart rate and the development of any arrythemias or conduction defects.(19)

Today, the step test has largely been replaced by the

bicycle ergometer, a stationary bicycle pedalled against increasing resistance, and the graded treadmill (Bruce Test), where one walks or jogs at varying speeds and exertion on an inclinable treadmill. Tables now exist that compare oxygen uptake values both at the submaximal level, as used for most post–heart attack patients, and at levels that are adjusted for age, weight, and sex. By comparing oxygen consumption value of a patient at a known exertion on the treadmill, a precise evaluation of the severity of cardiac impairment can be made. By subsequent testing after an interval of appropriate training, the patient can be retested and his aerobic gains (conditioning, representing increased pumping capacity of the heart) documented.

We use this concept of functional aerobic impairment to outline an appropriate exercise prescription. The aerobic impairment can be expressed as the percentage difference of submaximal or maximal oxygen consumption recorded for a patient, as compared to that figure predicted in health for a person of the same age, weight, and sex. The formula is:

$$\frac{\text{Predicted } VO_2 - \text{observed } VO_2 \text{ max}}{\text{predicted max } VO_2} \times 100$$

It is generally accepted that mild impairment is 27–40 percent, moderate 41–54 percent, marked 55–68 percent, and extreme over 69 percent.

Heart rate and body oxygen intake have a directly proportional or linear relationship at high submaximal and maximal levels of effort. For this reason, the heart rate itself can be used as a measurement of oxygen consumption. Tables are also available for the predicted heart rates for a given treadmill exertion for men and woman of various ages and weights. Thus, similar percentages can be obtained by applying the formula:

$$\frac{\text{Predicted heart rate} - \text{observed max. heart rate}}{\text{predicted max. heart rate}} \times 100$$

Using this method eliminates the need to collect and analyze oxygen concentrations in expired air.

Based on the results of exercise testing, the specific structure of the intensity, duration, and nature of the exercise work loads for the post–heart attack patient will be made. Training is aimed at increasing muscular flexibility and strength and aerobic performance. The end result of a training program for the post–heart attack patient depends on the level of fitness at the onset of training, genetic or inherited endowment, previous training, experience including the length of time and age at which the coronary occured, age, health, and the structure and duration of the training program.

What makes a conditioning program possible for heart attack patients is that they generally adapt to physical stress in a manner comparable to healthy, mildle-aged men and women. For the few whose stress exercise test is complicated by abnormal blood pressure, heart rate, or functional capacity, further medical treatment may be required before beginning an aerobic conditioning program.

What is Included in the Post–Heart Attack Exercise Prescription

For normal as well as heart attack patients, exercise prescriptions should consist of a comprehensive treatment program that affects all aspects of life and includes supervision and periodic re-evaluation. It should emphasize dieting to attain normal body weight and a reduction in saturated fats, abstinence from the use of tabacco, resumption of employment and normal social life, medication when necessary, and attention to psychological needs. Not only should the prescription build muscular strength and endurance, but it should be pleasurable and tailored to one's tastes as far as possible.

Most heart specialists concur (although there is some

disagreement) that the training session should last 30–60 minutes. In the beginning, they should be repeated at least three non-consecutive times per week—some physicians favor five. At least one study of post–heart attack patients, reported the same level of improvement with three exercise periods per week as with five, but it showed less progress for people who exercise fewer than three times a week.(15) For example, cutting back training sessions to once a week resulted in a 50 percent loss in aerobic performance over ten weeks. By stopping all exercise, this 50 percent loss occurred within five weeks.(24) Another study found all aerobic gains were lost in ten weeks if exercise stopped completely.(21)

As stated previously, all exercise programs should begin with a warm-up period, then include an intense workout, and finally end with a cooling-off phase. The intensity of the sessions can be revised on the basis of test re-evaluation or other illness or absenteeism.

Finally, both cardiac and normal patients should be aware of certain activities or conditions that modify training responses and may be potentially hazardous. They are:

1. Eating a large meal, especially one high in protein or fat, either two hours before, or within an hour of active exercise;
2. Drinking coffee, tea, or cola immediately before or after active exercise;
3. Drinking iced or very hot beverages, or any hard liquor during exercise;
4. Smoking at any time especially right after exercise;
5. Wearing heavy or poorly ventilated clothing during high-level sustained exercise;
6. Taking cold or very hot showers immediately before or after exercise;
7. Taking saunas, other than brief use of dry or wet "hot rooms";

8. Going quickly from a warm locker room to cold winter weather while still perspiring.

OBSERVATIONS OF EXERCISING POST-HEART ATTACK PATIENTS

Just as the endurance gains in the exercising post-heart attack patients are similar to those seen in other middle-aged Americans, so, too, are other benefits of regular exercise. I have previously commented on the alleviation of depression through exercise. In fact, most exercising heart patients report that they feel more energetic, are more productive, find work less boring, and have a more positive feeling about their health as well as their ability to deal with stress. Moreover, because of their exercise prescription, post-heart attack patients not only lose weight, but in general eat less and are more interested in weight control. Sleep is frequently sounder and more relaxed.

The exercise prescription therefore serves as a catalyst effecting a positive change in the heart attack victim's broad pattern of health behavior. In fulfilling the exercise prescription, they reflect on their state of health and what they can do about disease prevention and general health. Finally, the exercise prescription also serves to influence their feelings of health and well-being and self-esteem.

Now that you are more than two months past your coronary and have passed your stress EKG successfully, it's time to begin your exercise program. This step should be taken under the direction of your cardiologist. Your age, weight, condition you were in prior to your heart attack, and severity of your heart attack will determine both the initial level and the degree of progression of your exercise program. Acknowledging that there are various post-heart attack exercise regimens employed in cardiac rehabilitation centers, and that each exercise prescription should be tailored to the patient's unique requirements, the following is presented for you and your cardiologist's scrutiny.

A Sample First Year's Post–Heart Attack Exercise Program

First, some general points. Ultimately, the essential portion of your exercise program is the aerobic endurance phase. Initially, however, this part is deferred, as first the stomach and back are strengthened, and the entire body is conditioned, so that the aerobic phase can begin with little chance of injury. During the first year of this program, there is not the wide range of activities open to the non-heart attack individual. This is because, for the heart attack patient, it is important to know precisely the amount of work being done and the gradual increments. This eliminates sports, as the intensity of effort can vary too widely. Also, we want no added psychological stress—in this endeavor, everyone is a winner!

The Body Conditioner Phase. The first eight-week exercise program is outlined in Tables 7-1 and 7-2. In general, those who are over 45 or obese should begin with the regimen of Table 7-2. This is not a hard and fast rule though, and if your cardiologist feels you can safely start at the higher level, fine. For maximal benefits, these exercises should be done at least three times a week, and five times is recommended. The exercises are to be done consecutively, with rest periods of no more than two minutes. A sign of improvement in your level of fitness will be your ability to complete the sequence in a shorter period of time. Start slowly, gradually increasing the tempo. The exercises should never be done in a jerky manner, but rather, executed as smoothly as possible. They should be done in the sequence presented, as both a warm-up and

Table 7–1
Post–Heart Attack Body Conditioner Program for Those Under 45

Exercise	Repetitions	Description
1. Walk 3 minutes		1, p. 187
2. Bend and stretch	10	3, pp. 187–188
3. Rotate head	10 each way	4, p. 188
4. Body bender	5 increasing to 10	5, p. 188
5. Back flattener	5 increasing to 10	6, pp. 188–189
6. Wall press	5 increasing to 10	7, p. 189
7. Arm circles	5 increasing to 10	9, p. 190
8. Half knee bend	5 increasing to 10	10, pp. 190–191
9. Wing stretcher	5 increasing to 10	11, p. 191
10. Single knee hug	3 increasing to 10	14, p. 192
11. Single leg raise	3 increasing to 10	16, pp. 193–194
12. Straight arm and leg stretch	5 repetitions	18, p. 194
13. Heel-toe beam walk		20, p. 195
14. Knee push-up	2 increasing to 10	22, p. 196
15. Side leg raise	2 increasing to 10	23, p. 196
16. Advanced sit-up	2 increasing to 10	25, p. 197
17. Sitting bend	2 increasing to 5	27, pp. 198–199
18. Divers stance	hold 10 seconds	28, p. 199
19. Deep knee bend	2 increasing to 5	29, pp. 199–200
20. Walk 3 minutes		1, p. 187

cooling-off period are included in each series. A little stiffness should not deter your exercise plan, but frank pain that does not disappear in 48 hours means that that particular exercise should be deleted until it can be resumed without pain, or until medical clearance is given.

Of course, any chest pain, squeezing chest tightness, pain down the left arm, or unexplained trouble breathing signals an immediate stop to your exercises, a visit to your cardiologist, and his or her clearance before resumption of your program.

Table 7–2
Post–Heart Attack Body Conditioner Program for Those Over 45

Exercise	Repetitions	Description
1. Walk 2 minutes		1, p. 187
2. Bend and stretch	2 increasing to 10	3, pp. 187–188
3. Rotate head	2 increasing to 10 each way	4, p. 188
4. Body bender	2 increasing to 5	5, p. 188
5. Back flattener	2 increasing to 5	6, pp. 188–189
6. Wall press	2 increasing to 5	7, p. 189
7. Arm circles	5 each way	9, p. 190
8. Wing stretcher	2 increasing to 5	11, p. 191
9. Single knee raise	3 increasing to 10	13, p. 192
10. Straight arm and leg stretch	2 increasing to 5	18, p. 194
11. Heel-toe walk		19, p. 195
12. Side leg raise	2 increasing to 5	23, p. 196
13. Partial sit-up	2 increasing to 10	24, p. 197
14. Deep knee bend	2 increasing to 5	29, pp. 199–200
15. Walk	1 to 3 minutes	1, p. 187

For the first week, do the fewest repetitions or shortest duration of time shown for each exercise. If, after a week, you still find this level strenuous, do not increase the duration or repetitions. When you feel at ease with an exercise where a range of repetitions is given, slowly increase the number by one additional repetition per week, no faster. For those who have started with Table 7-2, if, after six or seven weeks you can easily do the entire series without resting between exercises, then you are ready to progress to Table 7-1. Before one leaves this body conditioner phase to progress to the advanced aerobics phase, one should be able to comfortably complete without rest periods the sequence of Table 7-1. Obviously, many who started at the lower level will not find this increase possible in eight weeks. It doesn't matter whether it takes eight or sixteen weeks, as long as safe, steady progress is realized.

The Advanced Aerobics Phase. Now that your body has firmed up, you are ready to safely engage in a more advanced aerobics phase. For the slender, either the walk-jog or bicycle riding program may be used. For the still-obese, depending on the degree of obesity, it may require a year or more of sensible dieting and exercise to attain your desired weight; for those with lower extremity orthopedic problems, the bicycle program is recommended.

Regardless of which of these two programs you pursue, the entire work-out should include a warm-up and cooling-off phase. It is suggested you select any three of the first ten exercises of Table 7-1 for your warm-up and any three of the last ten for your cooling-off period. Varying the selection on different days is recommended. As before, the minimal number of workouts per week is three, with five recommended.

For those pursuing the walk-jog program, it is recommended that you start at ½ mile. If you are not using a track, mark out with your car distances of .5 miles to 1.5

Table 7–3
Walk Time in Minutes

Week	Distance in Miles	Minutes (under 45 yr)	Minutes (over 45 yr)
1	0.5	9	10
2	0.6	10	11
3	0.7	11	12½
4	0.8	12½	14
5	0.9	14	15½
6	1.0	15½	17
7	1.1	17	18½
8	1.2	18½	20
9	1.3	20	21½
10	1.4	21½	23
11	1.5	23	25

miles in tenth-of-a-mile increments. Also, it is suggested that you invest in a good pair of training running shoes of correct width and length. While they are not essential for the walk phase, you will need them for jogging, and might as well be breaking them in from the beginning. As seen in Table 7-3, you are to increase the distance of your brisk walk one-tenth of a mile per week up to 1.5 miles. The time limits listed are to ensure a brisk pace, but never push yourself to the point of breathlessness.

By the start of the twelfth week, assuming you can comfortably finish the full mile-and-a-half distance in recommended time, you are ready to begin jogging. For those under 45, pace out fifty yards, (three wide steps equal one yard); for those over 45, pace out twenty-five yards. Start by jogging your twenty-five or fifty yards and then walking one hundred yards. Initially, jog at a rate just barely faster than your brisk walk. Then, slowly increase the speed to five m.p.h. as clocked by a car or bicycle speedometer. Gradually increase the jogging portion by about ten yards a week and reduce the walking segment a similar amount.

In about three months, most will be jogging about one-and-a-half miles. From this point on, add one-tenth of a mile per week up to two miles. When you can jog the full two miles in about twenty-five minutes, you have reached the minimum fitness level, one that probably far exceeds your condition prior to your heart attack.

Assuming you started this exercise program two months after your heart attack, it is now about ten months from that traumatic day. Over the next two months, it is suggested you add one-half mile every two weeks to your jogging. Thus, by the twelfth month you are jogging three to four miles. At this point, you are quite physically fit, and, with your doctor's permission, should be able to substitute any of the endurance activities of Table A-2 or Table A-4 in the Appendix for one of your three or more weekly workouts.

THE POST-HEART ATTACK SUPERACHIEVERS

If the jogging routine has become boring, it is permissible at this point to switch to one of the exercise programs found in Chapter 8 or 9. From previous experience at various cardiac rehabilitation centers, you have probably become hooked on running, and, if anything, may gradually increase rather than decrease your mileage.

As we have already mentioned, once the heart has healed from the initial infarction, most heart attack patients can expect to progress with an exercise program at a rate similar to those of other middle-aged Americans. This point was most dramatically made by a group of Toronto Rehabilitation Centre post-heart attack patients. Slowly and carefully trained and monitored by the center's director Dr. Terence Kavanaugh, this group unofficially entered and completed the prestigious Boston Marathon on Patriot's Day, 1973. This remarkable achievement so excited the Honolulu cardiologist, Dr. Jack Scaff, who directs a similar post-heart attack exercise program, that he introduced a special cardiac division into the First Honolulu Marathon held in December, 1973. Now five years later, nearly a thousand post-heart attack patients have increased their exercise programs to the point where they have safely completed full 26 mile 385 yard marathon runs. These feats are important as dramatic illustration of the value of the medically supervised post-heart attack exercise program. They point out just how far one's exercise prescription can be upgraded if one desires to put in the time and effort. But it is certainly not necessary to make such a commitment. A program just three to four hours a week is sufficient to gain the physiological and psychological benefits desired.

Those of you who still have more than 15 percent excess body fat at the completion of the body conditioner phase, could progress to the walk course, but I would not suggest jogging. This is because the excess weight produces unacceptable stress on your lower back, hips, knees, ankles, and feet. The chance of injury is unacceptable: over 50 percent. If your diet-exercise program does not have you at a near —desirable weight by the end of the three-month walk phase, plan instead to start on the bicycle program. When you reach the point of desirable weight in your bicycle program, you have the option of staying with your program or switching to the walk-jog regimen.

The bicycle program is less precise than the walk-jog, because the variability in types of bicycles and terrain must be considered. The same warm-up and cooling-off exercises apply, as does the frequency. Most can safely start at a distance of two miles. Try to cover this in twelve minutes or under, and maintain this level for the first month. Then, if you feel comfortable, add one-quarter of a mile a week over the next month. Before more mileage is added, increase your speed so that you can cover the three miles in fifteen minutes. As you again add mileage at about a half-mile per week, try to sustain the five-minute-per-mile pace. Hold the higher distance constant until it can be completed at that pace, then add another half-mile. This will become increasingly difficult with each addition. Your objective is to reach ten miles in fifty minutes or less. Bike riding will, thus, necessitate a longer exercise period to achieve a training effect comparable to jogging. *If at anytime you experience a dizzy, nauseated, seasick feeling, pain or tightness in your chest, or if your heart starts to pound, stop, walk home slowly, and check with your cardiologist before resuming your exercise program.*

For those who have no bike paths, trails, or suitable quiet streets on which to ride, and for those whose winters leave ice and snow on the ground, a stationary bicycle program can be substituted. A speedometer can reflect your speed and the distances adjusted similarily to the schedule just presented. Two comments are in order for the stationary biker. First, avoid the type of bike in which the handlebars go up and down like a rocking horse. Rather than producing more exercise, it creates an unacceptable imbalance on the foot pedal resistance. Second, most people honestly find this activity tedious. That can be alleviated somewhat by pedaling in front of the television or with the radio, stereo, or tape deck playing alongside. After you have reached your target distance and speed, ten miles in fifty minutes or less, and sustained it for a month, you may substitute one of the activities in Table A-2 or A-4 for one of your three-or-more weekly exercise periods.

FINAL REFLECTIONS FOR THE HEART ATTACK PATIENT

In this chapter, the values of a post–heart attack exercise program have been made quite clear. The benefits are far more than physical; there are emotional gains as well. Whereas such a program has been documented as reducing recurrent heart attacks, even if there were not an extension of life, the exercise program is fully justified by the markedly improved *quality of life.*

While several alternative post–heart attack exercise programs are presented in this chapter, I wish to conclude by repeating a warning stated earlier. Each heart attack is unique. The proper aerobic exercise prescription and its constant updating is also unique to the given individual. What is perfectly safe for one could be fatal for another. There is absolutely *no* place for you to attempt on your own an exercise program that has been made out for someone else. No matter how graphically the warning signals of chest pain, irregular or sudden rapid heart beat, or sudden or profuse sweating can be protrayed in a book, unless you are a cardiologist and can conduct your own exercise stress test, you have no business trying to outline or follow an exercise program alone. It is better not to undertake such a program at all than to do it without medical supervision.

8

Physical Fitness for Inactive Adults Under Sixty

Exercise.... is still the most potent antidote and prophylaxis against depression that we know. There is little doubt that depression heightens mortality. Excercise, therefore, is right on!

T. P. Hackett and N. H. Cassem, 1973

$\mathcal{T}$he importance of exercise for physical and spiritual health has long been recognized. As early as the seventeen hundreds, physicians and informed laymen in England, France, and Switzerland were writing on this subject.(17) However, only in the twentieth century has the need for physical exercise become critical. During the last twenty-five years, especially, American adults have assumed a primarily sedentary way of life. Earlier, hard physical labor in the house, shop, and field was an everyday necessity for both men and women; today, most of us spend our days in sedentary pursuits in the office, car, or in front of the television set. Therefore, the modern man and woman must consciously plan and follow an exercise program if he or she is to be physically fit.

Unfortunately, the vast majority of American men and women have *totally* neglected physical fitness. Many have not exercised to an appreciable extent since high school. Few can claim to have engaged systematically in any sustained exercise during the past five years. As a result, people 40 or older stand a much greater chance of contracting a major degenerative disease today than they would have twenty years ago or more. For example, even though newspapers have recently cited studies that suggest the incidence of fatal heart attacks has decreased, in reality this is not likely to be the case. These studies were based on death certificates filled out two decades ago when most medical examiners were political appointees, not doctors; and they listed virtually all non-traumatic sudden deaths as caused by heart attack. Today, autopsies are performed with much greater accuracy, and the true causes of death can be ascertained. More often than not, today's death certificates will list the cause of death as a "massive subarachnoid hemorrhage from a ruptured cerebral aneurysm," or "spontaneous intracranial hemorrhage," or "cerebral infaction," or "brain tumor with sudden hemorrhage or swelling."

To completely avoid the illnesses caused by sedentary habits, physical fitness should be a lifetime pursuit. the superbly conditioned athlete cannot afford to stop exercising after his or her competitive years, or they will soon lose the physical advantages they once had. In fact, former athletes tend to eat more than less sports-minded people and are more likely to gain weight unless they adopt new dietary habits upon retirement from competitive athletics.

Yet studies have shown that cardiovascular fitness can be attained at any age and even people who have never exercised regularly can become physically fit.(2) In addition, sex plays no role, and women can attain levels of fitness as quickly as men.(22)

What are the advantages of being physically fit? As we have already pointed out, an adequate fitness program increases cardiovascular function, reduces body fat, besides lowering resting and exercise heart rates, systolic blood pressure, and serum cholesterol.(22) These positive physical changes in response to an appropriate physical fitness program have been shown to occur in middle—aged men and women as well as males and females of any other age.(6, 14, 22)

But you cannot feel your blood pressure, pulse, or serum cholesterol; and while more energy and greater endurance is an obvious advantage of an exercise program, you may demand more. Well, there is more! Recent studies show that regardless of age, men and women who exercise are more intellectual, emotionally stable, self confident, and relaxed than their less fit friends. A bout of moderate exercise in middle-aged and older people serves as a natural tranquilizer, relieving anxiety and tension more than some drugs, such as Meprobamate, a commonly prescribed muscle relaxant-tranquilizer. In addition, habitual exercisers cope better with emotional stress than non-exercisers.(25) After sixteen weeks of training, a group of previously sedentary females between 35 and 52 years of age said that they felt "better, stronger, more energetic, enjoyed life more, and wished to continue with the exercise."

YOUR PHYSICAL FITNESS EXAMINATION

Before starting your exercise program let me urge that you should undergo a specialized medical examination. Most people mistakenly begin exercising without getting an adequate check-up first. If you are over 35, or have a family history of cardiovascular disease, or have experienced chest pain, you should definitely be examined. Even for people who do not fit these categories, a medical examination is desirable.

Unfortunately, many family physicians and even internists give inadequate pre-exercise examinations. For your own health safety, seek out a physician who's knowledgeable in aerobic exercising, whatever his primary specialty may be. The check-up should be comprehensive and include a family history of relevant medical problems and familial traits; a blood lipid profile; resting blood pressure; and a resting 12-lead electrocardiogram. Most importantly, the examiner should take an exercise 12-lead electrocardiogram. Only by stressing the heart in this way will latent arrythmias (irregular heart beats) and signs of heart strain be detected. Your doctor should also record maximal heart rate, that rate of exercise which leaves you totally out of breath, and associated blood pressure.

If heart irregularities appear, the exercise program will have to be greatly modified to avoid the risk of heart attack. Gradually, as your stress electrocardiogram improves, your level of physical conditioning can be advanced.

It is helpful, although not essential, to have your maximum oxygen uptake recorded. This test permits an objective comparison of a person's present level of fitness with age-related tables. It gives an accurate indication of an individual's present level of fitness and performance capability. Moreover, by retaking the examination at regular intervals after beginning an exercise program, a person can document his or her rate of physical fitness improvement.

While a test of maximal oxygen consumption (VO_2 max.) is the most precise measurement of one's fitness, several practical considerations render this test undesirable for all but the superbly conditioned athlete. First, since the endpoint is exhaustion, one must consider whether the subject quit short of exhaustion because of low tolerance to physical discomfort, lack of motivation, or even fear of a coronary. Because of these drawbacks, *sub-maximal oxygen consumption test* is the test most often used to determine fitness. It is based on the fact that oxygen consumption and heart rate both increase in a straight line in response to increased physical effort. Thus this test involves physical effort, usually either running on a treadmill or riding a bicycle ergometer, [that brings the heart rate up to 50 percent and then 75 percent of one's age-computed maximal level as read from tables.] Your maximal oxygen consumption is also measured at these two points and from these figures one can compute the VO_2 max. There is also a simple version of the sub-maximal test using tables which relate heart rate and oxygen consumption. Here one plots heart rate against workload and obtains a predicted VO_2 max. from a table of average equivalents, accurate within a range of 10 percent. This test eliminates the need to collect and analyze expired air and is therefore more practical in an office setting.

Finally, a complete exercise exam will include, although it is not essential, an assessment of body composition: lean body mass versus body fat. The only precise method of determining body fat is the immersion technique. Unfortunately, this test is usually unavailable except in certain exercise laboratories. However, an adequate alternative technique you can perform on yourself if you like, involves measuring your body fat at seven sites: behind the triceps muscle (back of the upper arm), at the inferior angle of the scapula, midaxillary (vertical skin fold on midaxillary line at the level of the fifth rib), suprailiac (vertical skin fold on the crest of the hip at the midaxillary line), abdominal (horizontal skin fold adjacent to the umbilicus), thigh (vertical fold on anterior thigh midway between hip and knee), and knee (vertical fold at the midpoint of the knee cap).(24) Use a caliper to measure the skinfold thickness in each area in millimeters, and then add up the total millimeters: this is your fat index. Repeat these measurements as your fitness schedule progresses. You can anticipate a 20 to 25 percent reduction in skinfold fat measurements even if you have not lost any total body weight. If dieting (see Chapter 2) is used in conjunction with exercise, then a much greater reduction of body fat can be expected. Since muscle weighs more than fat, it is possible to sustain your beginning weight during an exercise program and still lose considerable body fat. This is especially true for the non-overweight person. Those underweight may even experience a slight weight gain as muscle is added. Estimates of ideal weights for men and women over 25 are found in Tables 8–1 and 8–2.

YOUR OWN EXERCISE PROGRAM

Now that you have passed your physical examination, we can discuss the elements of your fitness prescription. Each exercise program should have three parts: a warm-up period, an endurance phase, and a cooling-off period. It is analogous to the race horse warming up, running the race, and returning to the paddock to be cooled off by walking.

The *warm-up* phase should be at least five minutes and include rhythmic, slow stretching movements of the trunk and limbs. This increases blood flow and stretches the postural muscles, preparing the body for sustained activity. This first stage is critical for the middle-aged person who has not exercised in several years. To ignore the warm-up is to risk muscle-pulls or more severe injuries. Table A-1 in the Appendix lists fourteen warm-up exercises, and you may choose any combination for your five minute warm-up period. Vary the exercises on different days to avoid monotony.

The *endurance* phase should last fifteen to thirty minutes. During this period, your cardiovascular system is stressed to increase aerobic capacity. To achieve maximal

Table 8-1
Ideal Weights for Men (Ages 25 and Over)

Height (with shoes)		Weight, lb (as ordinarily clothed)		
		Small Frame	Medium Frame	Large Frame
Ft	In.			
5	2	116–125	124–133	131–141
5	3	119–128	127–136	133–144
5	4	122–136	130–140	137–149
5	5	126–136	134–144	141–153
5	6	129–139	137–147	145–157
5	7	133–143	141–151	149–162
5	8	136–147	145–156	153–166
5	9	140–151	149–160	157–170
5	10	144–155	153–164	161–175
5	11	148–159	157–168	165–180
6	0	152–164	161–173	169–185
6	1	157–169	166–178	174–190
6	2	163–175	171–184	179–196
6	3	168–180	176–189	184–202

cardiovascular improvement, exercise vigorously enough during the endurance phase to be breathing at approximately 70 percent of your maximal aerobic capacity. This translates to 70 percent of your maximal heart rate. For most of us this means increasing our pulse rates to 120–140 per minute. You are breathing hard, but not falling into greater oxygen debt (gasping for air). As your aerobic capacity increases, you will also have to increase the time and intensity of the endurance phase in order to maintain the same 70 percent effort.

It was Dr. Kenneth Cooper, in his best selling books *Aerobics, The New Aerobics,* and *The Aerobics Way* who most successfully presented a readily understood method of quantifying exercise.(3, 4, 5) In his books, there are charts giving relative point values for different types of exercises. For example, swimming 250 yards in 5 minutes was worth 2 points, while playing handball for 30 minutes was worth 4½ points. It was Dr. Cooper's contention that, if one accumulated 30–34 points per week they could consider themself physically fit and expect a lowering of their blood cholesterol, blood glucose, blood triglycerides, body weight and fat, and systolic and diastolic blood pressure.

Dr. Cooper has very definite ideas as to what is essential to achieve total physical fitness. He summarized his research in two basic principles. First, if one exercises 12 - 20 minutes per day, it must be vigorous enough to sustain a heart beat of 140/minute. If the exercise is not that vigorous, to be equally beneficial it must be sustained for a longer period of time. Table 1–2, page 36, cites an example of some common exercise pursuits and their aerobic point value and caloric expenditure.

Table 8–2
Ideal Weights for Women (Ages 25 and Over)

Height (with shoes)		Weight, lb (as ordinarily clothed)		
		Small Frame	Medium Frame	Large Frame
Ft	*In.*			
4	11	104–111	110–118	117–127
5	0	105–113	112–120	119–129
5	1	107–115	114–122	121–131
5	2	110–118	117–125	124–135
5	3	113–121	120–128	127–135
5	4	116–125	124–132	131–142
5	5	119–128	127–135	133–145
5	6	123–132	130–140	138–150
5	7	126–136	134–144	142–154
5	8	129–139	137–147	145–158
5	9	133–143	141–151	149–158
5	10	136–147	145–155	152–166
5	11	139–150	148–158	155–169

Following five or six months of regular physical activity, you will be nearing an optimal training level, after which aerobic capacity gains tend to plateau. Only by sharply increasing the intensity and duration of your workouts, can you make further progress, which is unnecessary. Practically speaking, except for those competing in endurance sports, there is no physiological or psychological benefit in going beyond this. For most people, exercise three to four times per week is sufficient in the endurance phase. This permits adequate recovery between fitness sessions and prevents soreness and tiredness.

Which is the best endurance exercise for you? Some good exercises that can be used for the endurance phase include brisk walking, race walking, jogging, running, cycling, cross-country skiing, swimming, rope skipping, and bench or chair climbing (see Table A-2 in the Appendix). Whichever exercise you select, the primary emphasis should be on *safe* and *enjoyable* participation. Few will adhere to an exercise commitment that is not pleasurable. Therefore, do whatever you most enjoy. On those days when the weather is poor or when you cannot exercise in daylight, you may substitute indoor activities: jogging in place, walking stairs, or rope skipping.

The *cooling-off* phase is too often omitted in exercise. While the endurance phase significantly raises body temperature, increases the heart rate and blood pressure, and builds up lactic acid and other waste products in your muscles, the cooling-off phase allows the bodily functions to gradually return to normal and it helps to eliminate waste products from your muscles, minimizing the chance of stiffness and soreness the next day. The cooling-off phase should last at least five minutes and can last longer if desired. It should include gross body movements that emphasize range of motion of the joints. Calisthenics are ideal for this final step in your day's exercise program.

A proper fitness program for the person who has not exercised in five years may include the following activities performed at least three times weekly:

Warm-Up: Select any 3 exercises from Table A-2. Start with 3 repetitions and gradually increase to 10.

Endurance: Execute any 1 or 2 exercises from Table A-2 for 15–30 minutes, at a pulse rate of 120–140, or at an intensity that induces forced deep breathing.

Cooling Off: Do 5 minutes of any 3 exercises from Table A-3

As the tables suggest, the great advantage of this fitness program is that you can tailor it to your own likes and dislikes. Practically any vigorous physical activity can be used in the endurance phase, provided it is performed for a long enough period of time and with sufficient intensity. For example, a weekend ski trip or a vigorous tennis match can count for one of the required workouts. Or, you can substitute hard physical labor like snow-shoveling or sawing wood for one of the endurance periods. But whatever endurance exercise you choose, it should be performed at least three times weekly although there is nothing wrong with working out daily. For the diabetic, daily exercise is strongly recommended to achieve maximal control and prevention of vascular complications.(See Chapter 4.) If you become overly tired, however, reduce the time of the endurance activities in Table A-2 and spend more time on the exercises in Table A-1 and Table A-3.

FOR THE SUPERACHIEVER

Some of you may wish to push beyond the physical fitness program outlined above and enter competitive middle-aged athletics. Interest in competitive sports seems to go in cycles. Today jogging and long distance running races are experiencing a wave of popularity. Not so long ago, it was golf, then tennis. Television exposure is mainly responsible for the rollercoaster rise in popularity of golf and tennis. The rising interest in running has developed quite differently; except for the Oympics, it has had virtually no media exposure. Its popularity has come mainly from the ground swell of interest in physical fitness and the realization that it is one of the most effective means of attaining good health. An economical sport, with a good pair of running shoes the only essential expense, running is also a practical sport in terms of time spent. One can run almost anywhere, at almost anytime. For a modest expenditure, one can even run at night, wearing battery powered headlights that amply illuminate the road ahead, as well as warn oncoming cars and trucks. One word of caution, though, from personal experience: while these headlights provide enough light to see 10–20 yards in the distance, it is still very easy to get lost at night unless you are running on streets or paths that you know. I would advise you to do night-running only over a familiar course, as experimenting with new routes will almost guarantee getting lost.

The current interest in running extends beyond jogging. Recently, there has also been a surge of interest in long distance running. Both men and women are doing it.

The Boston Marthon is now so popular, that race officials have had to establish minimum qualifying times— times that would have meant a very respectable finish 25 years ago. Still, the official entry list exceeds seven thousand well-conditioned men and women. New races are springing up all over the country, with distances ranging from 6 to 26 miles.

In general, I believe long distance racing is a positive development in sports. Although an extreme form of exercise—change seems to evolve by extremes—it has awakened the American public to the advantages of physical conditioning. A word of caution, however, is warranted. Training for long distance races is definitely hazardous; the competitive runner lives with injury and pain. If your objective is to achieve physical fitness by running, it is not necessary to run long distance races. If you do enter races, try to avoid becoming competitive; rather, run at your own pace and enjoy the people, pageantry, and picturesque settings that accompany these "happenings."

Why not run competitively? Another reason is that a good runner is like a good tennis player; practice is essential, but the ability you were born with ultimately determines whether you rise much above the "hacker's" level. The idea that if I run the same 150 miles per week that Frank Shorter and Bill Rogers train, then I, too, can become an excellent runner, is simply hogwash! These are supremely gifted athletes. Most of us were not born with innate running speed, and no matter how much we improve our cardiovascular systems and strengthen our legs, the basic speed of foot will not be there, and our times will always be mediocre. Moreover, as mentioned above, long distance running can result in injury. It has been estimated that two-thirds of those training to race incur injuries serious enough to curtail running or require a doctor's examination. *Runners World* points out that, "50-mile-a-week runners are nearly twice as likely to be injured as those who run 25 miles a week," that, "Those who race are about twice as likely to get hurt as non-racers," and that, "Everyday runners are injured more often than those who take days off during the week." Thus, if the objective is physical fitness, it hardly makes sense to embark on a course likely to result in periods of enforced abstinence. For most, then, jogging, not competitive running, is the best means to physical fitness. It avoids both the chance of physical injury and the long, arduous work-outs that precede less-than-satisfying race results.

Now that I have presented the hazards of long distance running, let me close this chapter with some personal and practical realities. In general, men and women love competition and prefer a challenge. Having a goal to work toward gives zest and pleasure rather than boredom to work-outs. For example, my time for the Boston Marathon in 1977 was three hours forty-two minutes, twelve minutes too slow to qualify in my age group for next year's race. My goal then was to qualify for this race in 1978; I did so by increasing my training and running a marathon in Newport in three hours fifteen minutes. The point here is not that three hours fifteen minutes is a significant achievement; indeed the world class runners finished an hour ahead of me. Rather, the point is that I had set a realistic goal for myself—to run a marathon in less than three hours thirty minutes. For me the training in anticipation of this goal was as meaningful as the race itself. In fact, the outstanding virtue of long distance running is that everyone can be a winner! Just to complete a race is a thrill and ensures an excellent work-out. And only your own time need matter in terms of personal satisfaction. To your own self be true; and if you enjoy competition, you will always win in long distance running. However, let me caution you again that no one sport provides over-all physical fitness. An endurance sport such as long distance running or cross-country skiing provides only the endurance phase of your exercise prescription. The equally important warm-up and cooling-off exercises must be included in your day's work-out if your commitment to total fitness is to be achieved.

9

Fitness for the Aged: Why and How?

Exercise is good for both sexes, in every stage of life, but especially in childhood and old age.

Nicholas Andry (1723)

$\mathcal{T}$he November 1977 cover of *Runner's World* shows a picture of a smiling John A. Kelley, with arms outstretched, crossing the finish line of the Falmouth, 7.2 mile road race. The caption reads: "Will you look this alive on your 70th birthday?"(1) Since the life span of the average American male is about 67 years, you may even question being alive at 70. Yet the happiness in John's face and his lean muscular body testify to the positive effects of vigorous physical activity. John Kelley has run competitive races for a half a century. His first Boston Marathon was in 1928, and he has run more (forty-six) and finished more (forty-three) Boston Marathons than any other person. He won the event twice, in 1935 and ten years later in 1945, and holds seven age-group records. At 70, he continues to run about an hour a day on the roads or beach near his Cape Cod home. He races more than 15 times a year and says, "I'm still enjoying my training very, very much."

But, you say, "I am over 60 and have never vigorously exercised since my school years. I wish I had lived the life of John Kelley, but what can I possibly do now?" Well, today is the first day of the rest of your life. You will be a long time dead, but while alive, you are never too old to attain physical fitness! Take note of a 70-year-old patient who was evaluated medically just prior to his attempt to break the world age record for the mile—run. This man attended school through the 11th grade, but had never participated on any school teams or been involved with organized running. He worked forty years as a machinist. At the age of 60, he joined a YMCA exercise class and began with calisthenics and one mile of running each week. Gradually, he increased his running, and actually competed in the Boston Marathon for five consecutive years. Prior to his mile run, this elderly gentleman underwent exercise stress testing with oxygen uptake analysis, the objective testing of cardiovascular fitness. The oxygen consumption recorded was the highest ever achieved in his age group. On June 9, 1973, he ran in an AAU—sanctioned one mile race. His time, six minutes thirteen seconds, easily broke the age record of six minutes fifty five seconds, set in 1969. The former record holder, now 76 years young, finally had his record broken by an individual who had never seriously exercised until he was 60 years old!

Why cite these two over-65-year-old runners? Am I trying to turn all of you into serious runners? No, I am merely pointing out that if God gave you an unusually endowed body, you can resurrect it at almost any age short of the grave. Even if you are not so endowed, and 95 percent of the population of this country is not, you can still look forward to physical fitness and participation in athletics.

The retirement years should be happy ones, but only

those who are healthy, alert, and active can appreciate them fully. Yet, even if you enter your sixties with five decades of inadequate physical activity, you can still regain and maintain an active, lively way of life. Energy begets energy; the only way to increase your own level of energy is to increase your activity. To *keep* lively you must *be* lively!

This chapter presents a plan to increase your current level of physical fitness. How fit you become will depend upon the amount of movement you are willing and able to undertake. Research has shown us that cardiovascular fitness can be attained at any age. Furthermore, women advance as rapidly as men.

You may ask, "Why exercise in my final years?" The answer is found in the contention of most medical authorities that, regardless of age, exercise makes a person look, feel, and work better. Exercise stimulates the various bodily functions, especially the digestive process. It improves posture and through appropriate low back exercises it can eliminate low back pain and disability (see Chapter 5). Physical activity also reduces most coronary risk factors, including hypercholesterolemia, hypertension, and obesity. In addition, the well-conditioned person usually develops a positive self-image. Feeling more confidence in your body, you will be encouraged to thrust yourself into new and stimulating experiences. Instead of recovering from a fractured hip, you, as a physically fit elderly person, can look forward to a high degree of independence. Perhaps it is this quality of independence that is to be most prized in later years. The financial and psychological advantages are obvious: being able to plan and do things without leaning on relatives, friends, or paid help. To drive your own car, to succeed with do-it-yourself projects rather than paying someone else for the service, to go and come as you please, to be an asset rather than a liability in emergencies—these are forms of personal freedom well worth striving for.

The basis of physical fitness in later years, as at any age, is a fit cardiovascular system (see Chapter 1). In addition, in this age group, there are important exercises that specifically promote flexibility, coordination and agility, balance, muscular strength, and endurance. If they're not used, muscles grow soft and atrophy. The natural, slow decline of muscular strength and endurance can only be held off by keeping the muscles toned through regular exercise. So, too, the balance and equilibrium mechanisms of the body can be kept fit only through use; acclerated degeneration occurs with disuse. The tissue surrounding joints increase in thickness and lose their elasticity with advancing years. This process (and the same is true of arthritis) is greatly retarded by a daily exercise program that moves the joints through the full range of motion. Quite the opposite of prevailing notions, elderly people should be encouraged to bend, move, and stretch, as exercise will keep their joints flexible, muscles supple and springy, and heart feeling young.

To be of maximum benefit, the exercise program described below must be carried out daily—or nearly so. It should begin with a warm-up period including some easy stretching, pulling, and rotating movements. This will be followed by a period of vigorous physical activity which should be broken up by times of less strenuous exercise. Finally, the only way to improve your physical strength and conditioning is to systematically increase the physical work load. Once you can comfortably carry out a given physical exercise, say, five times, the next step is to do it six times ... and so on.

This same exercise principle applies to the conditioning of the cardiovascular-pulmonary system. To increase the efficiency of the heart and lungs, it is essential to perform continuous, rhythmic exercises long enough to stress the cardiovascular-pulmonary system. Thus, brisk walking, jogging, bicycling, cross-crountry skiing, for example, should be maintained until the body begins to perspire and the pulse rate rises above 130/minute for several minutes. Within ten minutes after exertion, your pulse rate should return to normal and you should not feel fatigued. If this does not occur, you are advancing too fast.

How to Determine Your Level of Fitness

What is a sensible exercise program for you? Obviously, this depends on your present health and level of cardiovascular fitness. It is recommended that you begin with a general physical examination and stress electrocardiogram. Hopefully, your physician is knowledgeable in aerobic exercising and can assist you in finding a starting point. However, if you do not have this luxury, you can determine your own level of fitness by several easy tests.

One way to check your fitness is the walk test. The intent of the walk test is to determine how many minutes, up to ten, you can walk briskly on a flat surface without experiencing undue shortness of breath or discomfort. If you can walk briskly for only three or fewer minutes, you are at level III. If you easily exceed three minutes, but cannot comfortably walk ten minutes, you are at level II. If you can easily walk ten minutes, then you may be at level I. To determine if you are level I, an additional test can be attempted with walking and jogging. Alternately, walk 50 steps and jog 50 steps for a total of six minutes. Walk at a rate of at least 120 steps per minute and jog at a rate of 144 steps per minute. If you must stop this test before six minutes have elapsed, you are at level II. If you can easily complete the six-minute test, you are at level I. For those who can complete 12 minutes of this test, you can move beyond level I to such exercises as jogging, swimming, cycling, and cross-country skiing (see Table A-2 in the Appendix).

To be of maximal value, these exercises should be done daily. A half hour should be sufficient time. Start easily, and slowly increase the tempo and number of repetitions. If you feel a little stiff do not let this deter you. However, if you experience frank pain that does not disappear in 48 hours, omit that exercise until it can be resumed without pain—or until medical clearance is given. The exercises for each level, I, II, and III, should be carried out in the sequence given, as both a warm-up and cooling-off period are built into each series. The cooling-off period has recently received much attention in the Olympic games. It has been shown (*Sports Medicine,* January 1977) that the cooling-off phase allows muscles to be drained of lactic acids, the products of anaerobic metabolism, and is the best way to prepare the body for strenuous activity the next day. If possible, keep a log or record of the exercises you perform, how many repetitions are done, and how much time was required. Many find doing the exercises to music makes them more enjoyable. Others find watching the evening news or listening to the radio while exercising relieves boredom. The exercises can be done alone, with family, or with friends. Clothing should be loose, comfortable, and quite stretchable rather than restrictive. Shoes should have no heels and non-skid soles.

Instructions for Level III (See Table 9-1)

You should attempt to complete the entire sequence of exercises without rest periods of more than two minutes. If necessary, though, take a longer rest period. An indication of improvement in your level of fitness will be your ability to complete the sequence in a shorter time period. Never carry out an exercise in a jerky manner to improve speed. All exercises should be done as smoothly as possible.

For the first week, do the fewest repetitions or shortest duration of time shown for each exercise. If, after a week,

Table 9-1

Your Own Exercise Program Based on Your
Level of Fitness: Level III

Exercise	Repetitions	Description
1. Walk 2 minutes		1, p. 187
2. Bend and stretch	2 increasing to 10	3, pp. 187–188
3. Rotate head	2 increasing to 10 each way	4, p. 188
4. Body bender	2 increasing to 5	5, p. 188
5. Back flattener	2 increasing to 5	6, pp. 188–189
6. Wall press	2 increasing to 5	7, p. 189
7. Arm circles	5 each way	9, p. 190
8. Wing stretcher	2 increasing to 5	11, p. 191
9. Single knee raise	3 increasing to 10	13, p. 192
10. Straight arm and leg stretch	2 increasing to 5	18, p. 194
11. Heel-toe walk		19, p. 195
12. Side leg-raise	2 increasing to 5 each leg	23, p. 196
13. Partial sit-up	2 increasing to 10	24, p. 197
14. 1 to 3 minutes— Alternate walk-jog		2, p. 187
15. Walk	1 to 3 minutes	1, p. 187

you still find this level requires a strenuous effort, do not increase the duration or repetitions. Only when you feel comfortable with an exercise where a range of repetitions is given, should you slowly increase the number by one additional repetition per week, no faster.

After you can execute the maximum number of repetitions indicated for each exercise, try to carry out the entire series without resting between exercises. When you can easily accomplish this, you are ready to move on to level II.

Table 9-2
Your Own Exercise Program Based on Your
Level of Fitness: Level II

Exercise	Repetitions	Description
1. Walk 3minutes		1, p. 187
2. Bend and stretch	10	3, pp. 187–188
3. Rotate head	10 each way	4, p. 188
4. Body bender	5 increasing to 10	5, p. 188
5. Back flattener	5 increasing to 10	6, pp. 188–189
6. Wall press	5	7, p. 189
7. Arm circles	5 increasing to 10	9, p. 190
8. Half knee-bend	5 increasing to 10	10, pp. 190–191
9. Wing stretcher	5 increasing to 10	11, p. 191
10. Single knee-hug	3 increasing to 10	14, p. 192
11. Single leg-raise	3 increasing to 10	16, pp. 192–193
12. Straight arm and leg stretch	5	18, p. 194
13. Heel-toe beam walk		20, p. 195
14. Knee push-up	2 increasing to 10	22, p. 196
15. Side leg–raise	2 increasing to 10 each leg	23, p. 196
16. Advanced sit-up	2 increasing to 5	25, p. 197
17. Sitting bend	2 increasing to 5	27, p. 198
18. Deep knee bend	2 increasing to 5	29, p. 199
19. 3 to 6 minutes— Alternate walk-jog		2, p. 187
20. Walk	1 to 3 minutes	1, p. 187

Instructions for Level II (See Table 9-2)

When you are ready for the level II exercise program, proceed in a manner similar to level III. Start at the fewest number of repetitions and gradually advance a repetition at a time until you are capable of performing the highest continuous number of repetitions of each exercise. When

Table 9–3

Your Own Exercise Program Based on Your
Level of Fitness: Level I

Exercise	Repetitions	Description
1. Alternate walk fifty steps and jog fifty steps for 3 min.		2, p. 187
2. Bend and stretch	10	3, pp. 187–188
3. Rotate head	10 each way	4, p. 188
4. Body bender	10	5, p. 188
5. Back flattener with legs extended	10	6, pp. 188–189
6. Wall press	5	7, p. 189
7. Posture check	5	8, p. 190
8. Arm circles	10 increasing to 15	9, p. 190
9. Half knee bend	10 increasing to 20	10, pp. 190–191
10. Wing stretcher	10 increasing to 20	11, p. 191
11. Wall push-up	10	12, p. 191
12. Double knee hug	3 increasing to 10	15, pp. 192–193
13. Single leg raise and knee hug	3 increasing to 10	17, p. 194
14. Straight arm and leg stretch	5	18, p. 194
15. Heel-toe beam walk		20, p. 195
16. Hop	5 on each foot	21, pp. 195–196
17. Knee push-up	5 increasing to 10	22, p. 196
18. Side leg raise	10 each leg	23, p. 196
19. Advanced modified sit-up	2 increasing to 10	26, p. 198
20. Sitting bend	5 increasing to 10	27, pp. 198–199
21. Divers stance	hold 10 seconds	28, p. 199
22. Deep knee bend	5 increasing to 10	29, pp. 199–200
23. 5 minutes alternate walk-jog		2, p. 187
24. Walk	3 minutes	1, p. 187

this can be accomplished without straining or undue fatigue, you are ready to advance to level I.

Instructions for Level I (See Table 9-3)

The same directions, starting with the fewest repetitions and gradually increasing to the maximum number without rest periods, is to be adhered to. When you can perform the maximum without rest periods, you can either continue to increase the number of repetitions and speed of their execution, or advance to other, more vigorous exercises and sports i.e., jogging increasingly greater distances, swimming progressively longer distances, cross-country skiing, or any of the sports in the light or light moderate group of Table A-7 in the Appendix.

As we have previously discussed, this fitness program should ideally be completed in thirty minutes. Once you can accomplish this, you are ready to substitute what may be more enjoyable and more productive exercises. If you enjoy sports, then you may substitute, on any given day, 15 minutes of a maximal exercise sport, i.e., running, stationary running, cycling, cross-country skiing, or swimming (see Table A-2); or substitute thirty minutes of moderate sports activity, i.e., tennis, skiing, etc. (See Table A-7); or 45 minutes of minimal exercise sports, i.e., golf, gardening, canoeing, bowling, fishing, archery, horseshoes, Ping Pong, shuffleboard, or social dancing (see Table A-7).

Just as sports can be graded into maximal, moderate, and minimal exercise and energy output, a number of household projects can also be graded and substituted for the exercise program. In the maximal exercise group, some of these would include chopping wood, shoveling snow, and digging holes; in the moderate group, mopping and/or scrubbing a floor, gardening such as pushing a lawn mower, digging and pulling weeds; in the minimal exercise group, sweeping floors, ironing, washing clothes, making beds, light gardening.

However, the single easiest way to increase physical activity is simply to walk whenever possible. Once you have attained level I fitness, then the elevator should be obsolete for less than three floors and you should also park the car and walk at every chance.

Once you have successfully completed your fitness program in 30 minutes, you may substitute 30–60 minutes of any single or combined activity from Table A-4, 60–90 minutes of activity from Table A-5, or an hour or more of activity from Table A-6.

When carrying out the sequence of exercises outlined for levels I, II, or III, the order includes a warm-up, an endurance, and a cooling-off phase. The warm-up and cooling-off periods should not be forgotten when substituting other activities for the specific exercise routines. Five minutes of any exercise from Table A-1 should preceed your substituted activity and five minutes of exercise from Table A-3 should follow it.

Inevitably, some people who have attained level I fitness will seek more vigorous endurance activity. Many men and women in their sixties and seventies have taken up jogging two miles or more daily. This is to be applauded, but do not substitute jogging for your entire exercise program. While a splendid cardiovascular exercise, it does nothing for upper body muscle tone or joint flexibility and mobility. Jogging should always be preceeded by stretching exercises and in addition, calisthenics and other conditioning exercises listed in level I must be included if you are to achieve a balanced and complete work-out.

After jogging, you should cool off with five minutes of walking or five minutes of exercises from Table A-3.

Several additional points on jogging are especially pertinent to an older population. First, if you jog, you *must* wear appropriate running shoes. Basketball shoes, sneakers or deck shoes will not suffice. Specially constructed running shoes provide foot and arch support and have multi-layered flat non-skid soles that cushion the force of impact as you land on your feet. Unlike tennis shoes that do not have widths, good running shoes come in a variety of widths, and extreme care is essential in obtaining a precise fit. Most podiatrists recommend trying on shoes at the end of the day when your feet have swollen to their maximum size.

Second, when jogging, wear soft, loose-fitting clothing. Tight-fitting or abrasive clothing, heavy from perspiration, will chafe the skin, especially the nipples, groin, and axilla. It is seldom too cold to jog if you wear adequate clothing. This includes gloves and a hat or cap with adequate ear protection. Only a high wind-chill factor should force you to exercise indoors, as jogging then may result in frostbite. Also, never jog on ice or other slippery surfaces.

While in winter it is rarely too cold to jog unless the wind-chill factor is high, in summer it is often too hot. Do not jog at mid-day, especially when temperatures and humidity are high. And replenish lost body fluids promptly, either during or after your warm weather workout.

Nighttime jogging is also dangerous as you may stumble and fall. Only if a running area is adequately illuminated, like at a lighted track, or by wearing a headlight, should you jog at night, and only then over known, flat surfaces.

To conclude this chapter, let me mention two exercises —swimming and cross-country skiing—that are nearly perfect for the whole body. Unlike jogging, which does little to strengthen or increase upper body joint flexibility, they each combine a vigorous cardiovascular endurance workout while strengthening and increasing flexibility of nearly all joints. Both are highly recommended as a substitution or addition to your regular exercise program.

Finally, let me state again the risks of competing in sports as opposed to following a personal fitness program. Competition should be avoided if the primary objective is physical fitness, as competition will invariably bring a stress-related injury resulting in an enforced layoff. However, for some, myself included, the stimulus of competition makes otherwise tedious exercise tolerable. Training that is not directed toward a specific objective is difficult to maintain. Also, there is a special joy in competing, whether against an opponent in tennis or against the clock in long distance running. In distance races, so many people usually enter that, except for three or four in each class, the remainder are running against their previous best time. By retaining the common sense never to extend yourself too far in competition, its rewards will overshadow any minor injuries you may incur. However, no one should allow participation in one sport to replace his or her total exercise program.

10

Conclusion

Fortune is the arbiter of half the things we do, leaving the other half or so to be controlled by ourselves.

Niccolo Machiavelli (1469–1527)

*T*he intent of this book has been to present a no-nonsense, feet-on-the-ground rather than head-in-the-clouds approach to an intelligent physical fitness program for adults. It has not been written for the "weekend jock," but rather, for the majority of adults who, like myself, are not the "healthy elite." I have presented exercise programs specifically tailored to your medical problem(s), be it diabetes, a heart attack or coronary condition, obesity and/or hypertension, low back pain, a stroke, spinal cord injury, amputation or other physical disability, simple inactivity for five years or more, or just advanced age.

With each exercise regimen, except for the post–heart attack patient where initially precise monitoring of workloads and avoidance of psychological stress is mandatory, you have been given a wide range of physical activities, leisure and recreational pursuits, with which to compose your own exercise prescription. Thus, your personal tastes, work patterns, and lifestyle are taken into consideration whenever possible.

I have attempted in the cardiovascular chapter to give you a basic understanding of how and why cardiovascular disease occurs, and how vigorous, aerobic three-times-a-week or more physical activity may retard the process. What constitutes physical fitness, the efficiency of our cardiopulmonary system as measured by our ability to consume oxygen, is discussed in basic, practical terms. The concept of our own "biologic clock," our individual genetic endowment which translates into a potential fixed period of time on earth, is presented. While this "ideal physiological lifespan" is certainly important to a lengthy productive life, of even greater significance is the fact that we not speed up our "biologic clock." It is shocking, tragic, and economically costly the way most of us, by inappropriate life habits (i.e., self-pollution with excess food, alcohol, drugs, cigarette smoking, and simple physical inactivity) rob ourselves out of years or even decades of good health and life itself.

Also in this book, you are introduced to the myriad physiological and equally important emotional benefits derived from aerobic endurance exercise and the attainment of physical fitness. The mechanisms and health implications of the positive influences of aerobic physical exercise on our blood vessels and body chemistry, heart, lungs, glandular (endocrine) function, and emotions are detailed. Far from just the most commonly known effects of such exercise, slowing of the heart rate, increased functional capacity of the lungs during exercise, reduction in body fat and blood cholesterol, and a reduction in the tendency for depression, strain, and nervous tension resulting from psychological stress, a total of thirty-five positive health influences are covered.

In the chapter on nutrition, I have covered the essentials of what a good diet is, and how it should be modified for the vigorously exercising adult. I have discussed the cholesterol hypothesis from its conception in 1808 to the very latest controversy raised by Dr. George Mann's recent article in the *New England Journal of Medicine.* The facts known, theories proposed, and pure myths about vitamins are explored, including the present vitamin B$_6$–homocysteine hypothesis as regards arteriosclerosis. How the composition of our diet (i.e., degree of saturated fats, fiber content, salt, refined sugar, etc.) affects caloric intake and predisposition to various disease states is discussed and appropriate recommendations are made.

The presence of excessive body weight places significantly increased stress on your low back, hips, knees, ankles, and feet. That fact necessitates an exercise regimen for the obese that alleviates the problem. The injury rate for the obese who take up jogging is unacceptably high, well over 50 percent. Thus, specific aerobic exercise programs for the still-obese are outlined in this chapter— exercises that can be carried out seated or in water. The essential synergy between exercise and diet is discussed, as is the concept of weight maintenance being integrated early in your dietary regimen. It is not just the loss of weight that is important, but the accumulation of dietary habits and regular exercise that will ensure lifelong weight control.

The diabetes chapter is perhaps more comprehensive than necessary for the message imparted: *exercise is mandatory for maximal control of your disease, and daily exercise will likely retard the development of vascular complications.* Furthermore, the cardiovascular system of the diabetic can become conditioned as quickly as that of the non-diabetic. There is virtually no exercise pursuit the diabetic need avoid, and hypoglycemia with sustained exercise over forty minutes in duration is the only significant risk factor. Means to avoid this possible event by adjusting pre-exercise carbohydrate intake and/or insulin administration is fully discussed, as is how to handle a hypoglycemic reaction. Other exercising tips from the site of insulin administration to foot care are covered.

The metabolism of exercise in the diabetic and nondiabetic is compared and the role of exercise on liberalizing carbohydrate intake explained. The stages of diabetes, prediabetes, chemical diabetes, and overt diabetes are each explained as is the role of obesity in adult-onset diabetes.

This chapter was not only prepared from a comprehensive review of the literature on this subject, but also information gained from detailed questionaires from fourteen diabetic marathoners, as well as the invaluable experience of living and sharing one's life with an exercising diabetic, my wife Jane.

Next to dental caries and the common cold, low back pain is one of our most common physical afflictions. Virtually all of us will suffer with this malady at one time or another. As someone who has incurred this affliction and overcome it to a degree that competitive long-distance running and tennis are presently enjoyed, and, as a neurosurgeon who sees over one hundred people monthly with this problem, this chapter has a very personal basis for me. While it is true that surgery is unavoidable for a small percentage of people with back pain, primarily those with large ruptured discs with a neurological deficit that does not clear with prolonged conservative treatment, or cases of progressive spinal instability, most, like me, can be returned to full, vigorous activity with the exercise program, do's and don't's, outlined in this chapter. Once your back problem is overcome, you are urged to progress to a suitable fitness program as outlined in either Chapter 8 or 9.

The chapter on fitness for the physically disabled proved inspiring for me to research and write. Professionally, I am daily reminded of the severe neurological impairments that can befall us without a moment's warning. And while I am very familiar with prescribing the various inhospital physical therapies, I was almost overwhelmed with the recreational pursuits enjoyed by this group. With special equipment and other modifications, the physically disabled enjoy all sports from archery to wrestling, scuba diving to sky diving. The same physical and perhaps heightened emotional benefits are derived from exercise by the disabled as by those of us not so afflicted. As shown by the exercise programs in this chapter, they too, require warm-up, endurance, and cooling-off phases to their exercise regimens. Special programs are outlined for the upper limb, lower limb, and both upper and lower limb disabled.

For the superachievers, the disabled can enter their own national and international competitions—including a special olympics for the handicapped. I sincerely hope the athletic organizations for the disabled and the selective bibliography of recreational activities for the handicapped presented at the end of this chapter will be enthusiastically received and used.

The post–heart attack chapter was not written without considerable soul-searching on my part. While throughout it I continually plea that you not undertake the exercise regimen except under a cardiologist's direction, I know some of you will not heed my advice. This is unlike an occasional patient of mine who, to avoid paying for an office visit, will call me on the day of an appointment stating they have transportation problems ... and by the way, what did the latest tests show and how do I want them to adjust their medication in the future; I can usually safely conduct this gratis "office non-visit" over the phone. To attempt to undertake a post–heart attack exercise program without medical supervision and periodic updating of cardiac status could save you a few dollars, *but prove fatal. Please do not take this risk.* Exercise testing is explained in detail as are the latest concepts in post–heart attack care and rehabilitation. Tips on potentially hazardous activities are listed as well as the reason why cigarette smoking for the coronary patient is suicide. Finally, two precise postcoronary exercise programs are detailed in this chapter, one for the slender and one for the still overweight.

Perhaps, most who buy this book or receive it from a friend or family member will fall into the group of physically inactive for five or more years. While the virtues of exercise for physical and spiritual health were prevalent in the medical and lay writings of seventeenth century Europe, only during the twentieth century has the need for physical exercise become critical. Whereas we formerly received adequate exercise from our daily routine, in the past half-century, with urban migration, invention of the car and other forms of mass transportation, and mechanization of our daily activities at home and at work, we now must actually plan our exercise. Indeed, in medicine today, we have an entire new grouping of diseases called *hypokinetic* illnesses which are directly the result of physical inactivity.

In this chapter, you are given the basics of a physical fitness examination, then presented the information necessary to construct and update your own comprehensive exercise program. To the superachievers, appropriate warnings are given, but no water thrown on the fire.

It was Nicholas Andry, in the early seventeen hundreds, who wrote, "Exercise is good for both sexes, in every stage of life, but especially in childhood and *old age.*" In the fitness for the aged chapter, it is made quite clear that the basis of physical fitness at any age is a fit cardiovascular system. While exercise programs for our senior citizens should specifically promote flexibility, coordination, agility, balance, and muscular strength, aerobic endurance exercise is still primary. After you have been instructed in how to determine your level of fitness, you are directed to proceed to one of these appropriate, comprehensive programs. Progression from one level to another as fitness increases is carefully detailed, as well as the point up to where any physical pursuit can safely be enjoyed.

In closing, it is my most sincere desire that after reading your selected parts, and, hopefully, the entire book as well, that you will feel its intent, as expressed in the opening sentence of this chapter, has been realized.

Appendix: Exercises

Table A–1

Warm-Up Exercises

Exercise	Description
1. Back flattener	6, pp. 188–189
2. Single knee raise	13, p. 192
3. Single knee hug	14, p. 192
4. Double knee hug	15, pp. 192–193
5. Single leg raise	16, pp. 193–194
6. Partial sit-up	24, p. 197
7. Advanced sit-up	25, pp. 197–198
8. Sitting bend	27, pp. 198–199
9. Deep knee bend	29, pp. 199–200
10. Posture check	8, p. 190
11. Bend and stretch	3, pp. 187–188
12. Wall push-up	12, p. 191
13. Hop 3 min.	21, pp. 195–196
14. Divers stance	28, p. 199

Table A–2
Endurance Exercises

1. Badminton
2. Basketball
3. Bench or stair climbing
4. Boxing
5. Canoeing
6. Continuous vigorous passing of a medicine ball
7. Continuous vigorous pulling of weights from a wall pulley system
8. Cycling
   A. Stationary
   B. Moving
9. Dancing
   A. Ballet
   B. Fast social
   C. Square
   D. Tap
11. Handball
12. Jogging
    A. In place
    B. Moving
13. Paddle tennis
14. Rope skipping
15. Rowing a single scull or a machine
16. Running
17. Skiing
    A. Cross country
    B. Downhill
    C. Water
18. Skating
    A. Ice
    B. Roller
19. Skindiving
20. Squash
21. Swimming
22. Touch football
23. Walking uphill or in sand or water

Table A–3
Cooling-Off Exercises

Exercise	Description
1. Walking 5 min.	1, p. 187
2. Alternate walk-jog 3 min.	2, p. 187
3. Rotate head	4, p. 188
4. Body bender	5, p. 188
5. Wall press	7, p. 189
6. Arm circles	9, p. 190
7. Half knee bend	10, pp. 190–191
8. Wing stretches	11, p. 191
9. Single leg raise and knee hug	17, p. 194
10. Straight arm and leg stretch	18, p. 194
11. Heel-toe walk	19, p. 195
12. Heel-toe beam walk	20, p. 195
13. Knee push-up	22, p. 196
14. Side leg raise	23, p. 196

EXERCISES

1. *Walk (3 Minutes)*

Objective. An excellent warm-up exercise to loosen muscles and prepare you for the ensuing exercises.

Basic Exercise. Stand erect, be well balanced on the balls of your feet. Begin walking rapidly on a level surface.

2. *Alternate Walk-Jog (3 Minutes)*

Objective. Warm-up exercise for more advanced exercises; good for legs and circulation.

Basic Exercise. Stand erect as for walking, with arms held flexed and forearms roughly parallel to the floor. Begin by walking for 50 steps, then break into a slow run (jog) for 50 steps. When jogging, stride easily, landing on your heels and rolling to push off on your toes. This heel-toe movement is in contrast to a fast run, where you land and stay on the balls of your feet. Arms should swing freely from the shoulders in opposition to the legs. Breathing should be deep, but never labored to the point of gasping. Continue for 3 minutes.

3. *Bend and Stretch*

Objective. To loosen and stretch primarily the back, hamstring, and calf leg muscles.

Basic Exercise. Stand erect with your feet shoulder-width apart. Slowly bend forward at the waist and touch the fingers of your outstretched arms to your toes, bending your knees to whatever degree is necessary to accomplish this maneuver. The maximal effort is achieved when the knees can remain locked. Return slowly and smoothly to the starting position.

4. Rotate Head

Objective. To loosen and relax muscles of the neck and firm up the throat and chin line.

Basic Exercise. Stand erect with your feet shoulder-width apart and your hands on your hips. Slowly, use a smooth motion to rotate your head in a full circle from left to right; then slowly rotate your head in a full circle from right to left.

5. Body Bender

Objective. To stretch arm, trunk, and leg muscles.

Basic Exercise. Stand erect with feet shoulder-width apart and your hands extended overhead with your fingertips touching, as in a praying hand posture. Slowly bend sideward at the waist as far to the left as possible while keeping your hands together and your arms extended straight. Return to starting position; repeat same movements to the right.

6. Back Flattener

Objective. Strengthen gluteal (buttock) and abdominal muscles and flatten the low back, lumbar lardosis.

Basic Exercise. Lie on your back on a padded floor with knees well bent. Relax, with arms above your head. (A small pillow may be placed under your head if desired.) Now squeeze your buttocks together as if trying to hold a piece of paper between them. At the same time suck in and tighten the muscles of your abdomen. You should feel your back flatten against the floor. This is the *flat back position*. Hold this position for a count of ten (10 seconds), relax and then repeat the exercise three times in the beginning. Gradually attempt to increase to 20 repetitions.

Advanced Modifications

BUTTOCK RAISE.   After the basic exercise has been done for a week or more, additional flattening can be achieved by doing the exercise with the buttocks slightly raised (1 to 2 inches) off the floor at the time the buttocks are squeezed and abdomen tensed. Hold for the count of ten, relax and repeat.

LEGS EXTENDED.   After several weeks of the basic exercise, gradually do the exercise with the knees less and less bent, until you can execute the exercise with your legs straight. The buttock raise need not be combined with this modification.

7. Wall Press

Objective.   To promote good body alignment and posture while strengthening abdominal muscles.

Basic Exercise.   Stand erect with your head and neck in a loose position, your back against the wall, and your heels 3 inches away from the wall. Suck in your stomach and press your low back flat against the wall. Hold this position for six seconds, relax, and return to the starting position. Your low back should continually be in contact with the wall and your head and neck should not extend backward.

8. Posture Check

Objective. To help you stand and walk correctly. To help you in determining if your exercise program is accomplishing its goals.

Basic Exercise. Stand with your back to the wall pressing your heels, buttocks, shoulders and head against the wall. You should be unable to feel any space between your low back and the wall—if you can, your back is too arched and not flat. Move your feet forward, bending your knees so your back slides a few inches down the wall. Now again squeeze your buttocks and tighten your abdominal muscles flattening your lower back against the wall. While holding this position, walk your feet back so you slide up the wall. Now, standing straight, walk away from the wall and around the room. Return to the wall and back up to it to be certain you've kept the proper posture.

9. Arm Circles

Objective. To strengthen the muscles of the shoulder while keeping the joint flexible.

Basic Exercise. Stand erect with your arms outstretched sideward at shoulder height, palms up. While keeping your head erect, make small circular movements with your hands backward as if describing a perfect circle: then reverse with your palms down, and carry out the circular movements in a forward direction.

10. Half Knee Bend

Objective. To strengthen and stretch your quadraceps (upper front thigh) muscles while improving your balance.

Basic Exercise. Stand erect with your hands on your hips. While extending your arms forward, palms down, bend your knees halfway. Keep your heels on the floor, pause and return to the starting position.

11. Wing Stretcher

Objective. To strengthen the muscles of the upper back and shoulders while stretching the chest muscles and promoting good posture.

Basic Exercise. While standing erect, bend your arms in front of your chest with your elbows at shoulder height and your extended finger tips touching. Count 1, 2, 3; on each count, pull your elbows backward as far as possible while keeping your arms at shoulder height and then returning to the starting position. Then, on the count 4, swing your arms outward and sideward, shoulder height, palms up, and return to the starting position. As you do this exercise count to yourself one and two and three and four . . .

12. Wall Push-up

Objective. Strengthen arm, shoulder, and upper back muscles while stretching chest and posterior thigh muscles.

Basic Exercise. Stand erect, squarely facing the wall, with your feet about six inches apart and arms extended straight in front of you with your palms on the wall lightly bearing weight. Slowly bend your elbows and lower your body towards the wall turning your head to the side until your cheek almost touches the wall. Then slowly push away from the wall, extending your elbows while returning to the initial position. Slowly repeat, this time turning your head to the opposite side.

13. Single Knee Raise

Objective. Stretch low back, hip flexor, and hamstring (posterior thigh) muscles.

Basic Exercise. Lie on your back on a padded floor with your arms above your head and your knees bent. Tighten your buttocks and abdominal muscles as in exercise No. 6. Then raise one knee over your chest toward your chin as far as possible, hold for ten seconds, return to starting position, and relax a few seconds before repeating with the opposite leg. Start with three repetitions of each knee, gradually advancing to ten.

14. Single Knee Hug

The single knee hug is essentially the same exercise as the single knee raise, except the hands are not placed above the head, but rather, are placed around the knee to be raised. The arms are used to pull (raise) the knee higher over the chest than was possible in exercise No. 13. This produces greater stretching of the low back and hamstrings.

15. Double Knee Hug

Objective. Stretch low back and hamstring muscles, strengthen abdominal and hip flexing muscles.

Basic Exercise. Lie on your back on a covered floor with knees bent, arms at your side, and pillow under your head, if desired. Tighten your buttocks and abdominal muscles so that your low back is flat against the floor. Now grasp both knees with your hands and raise them slowly over your chest as far as possible. Hold ten seconds, return to starting position, relax a few seconds, then repeat. Start with three repetitions and gradually build to ten.

Advanced Modification. After a month or more of the basic exercise, attempt the double knee hug starting with both legs extended straight. Tense your buttocks and abdomen and then taking care to keep the back flat, bend both knees, grasp knees with hands and raise over your chest, hold ten seconds and return to starting position to relax before repeating. The low back tends to arch when lifting and lowering the knee. If you cannot do this with your back against the floor, you are not yet ready for this modification and should resume the basic knees bent position. This extended leg starting position strengthens both the hip-flexing and abdominal muscles.

16. Single Leg Raise

Objective. Stretch low back and hamstring muscles, strengthen abdominal and hip-flexing muscles.

Basic Exercise. Lie on your back on a covered floor with one knee bent and one leg straight, arms at your side and a pillow under your head, if desired. Tighten your buttocks and abdominal muscles, then slowly raise the leg keeping it straight and your back flat. Raise the leg as far as comfortably possible, then slowly lower the leg, keeping it straight and your back flat, to the floor. Relax a few seconds and then repeat with the other leg. Start with three repetitions of each leg and gradually increase to ten.

Advanced Modification. After a month or more, attempt the single leg raise starting with both legs extended straight. Tense your buttocks and low back, and with your back flat and legs out straight, raise one leg up as far as possible. As the leg is raised, your back may not remain flat. Check by using your hand to see if your back lifts from the floor when the leg is lifted and lowered. If it does, resume the basic exercise with one knee bent.

17. Single Leg Raise and Knee Hug

Objective. Strengthens low back and abdominal muscles, while increasing flexibility of hip and knee joints.

Basic Exercise. Raise extended left leg about 12 inches off the floor, slowly bend your knee and move it toward your chest as far as possible using your abdominal, hip, and leg muscles: then place both hands around your knee and pull it slowly toward your chest as far as possible; slowly extend your leg to the position 12 inches off the floor; return to the starting position. Repeat 2 to 5 times with each leg. Do the number desired with the left leg, then switch and repeat with the right leg.

18. Straight Arm and Leg Stretch

Objective. Strengthens abdominal muscles while stretching the muscles of the arms.

Basic Exercise. Lie on your back, legs extended, feet together, arms at your side, your buttocks and abdomen tensed so your back is flat against the floor. Slowly move arms and legs outward along the floor as far as possible, hold a moment and slowly return to the starting position. Repetitions as indicated for each level.

19. Heel-Toe Walk

Objective. To improve balance and posture.

Basic Exercise. Stand erect with abdomen and buttocks tensed, your left foot along a straight line and your hands held out from your body to aid in balance. Walk ten steps along the straight line by placing the right foot directly in front of the left with the right heel touching the left great toe, then alternating feet, placing the left in front of the right, heel-to-toe. When ten such steps in a straight line have been taken, stop; then return to the starting position by walking backward along the same line, alternately placing one foot behind the other, toe-to-heel.

20. Heel-Toe Beam Walk

Objective. To improve balance and posture.

Basic Exercise. Level II will walk ten steps on a 2 inch high by 6 inch wide board placed flat on the floor, level I, on a 2 inch high by 4 inch wide board placed flat on the floor. Walk ten steps along the board by placing the right foot directly in front of the left with the right heel touching the left great toe, then alternating feet placing the left foot in front of the right, heel-to-toe. When ten such steps have been taken, stop, then return to the starting position by walking backward along the same board alternately placing one foot behind the other, toe-to-heel.

21. Hop

Objective. To improve balance, strengthen the extensor muscles of the leg and foot, and increase circulation.

Basic Exercise. Stand erect, low back flat, with your weight on your right foot and your left leg bent at the knee, your left foot several inches off the floor; hold your arms slightly outward from your body to aid in balance. Hop five times on your right foot and then hop five times on your left foot.

22. Knee Push-up

Objective. To strengthen the muscles of your arms, shoulders, and trunk.

Basic Exercise. Lie on the floor with your face down, legs together, knees bent with feet off the floor and your hands palm down flat on the floor under your shoulders. Slowly push your upper body off the floor extending your arms fully and keeping your low back flat so your body is in a straight line from head to knees. Slowly return to starting position, then repeat.

23. Side Leg Raise

Objective. To improve the flexibility of the hip joint and strengthen the lateral muscles of the trunk and hip.

Basic Exercise. Lie on the floor on your right side, with your head resting on your right arm and both legs extended together. Lift your top (left) leg off the right leg as far as possible. Stop, then return to the starting position and your left side and repeat the exercise with your right leg.

24. Partial Sit-up

Objective. Strengthen low back and abdominal muscles.

Basic Exercise. Lie on your back on a covered floor with your knees well bent and arms extended flat over your head. Squeeze your buttocks and tighten your abdominal muscles; with your low back on the floor, slowly raise your head, neck, and lastly shoulders as you extend your arms to your knees. Keep your low back flat on the floor. Hold this position ten seconds, then return to starting position, rest a few seconds and repeat. Start with three repetitions and progress to at least ten.

Advanced Modification. After you have progressed to ten repetitions, begin to progressively lift your head and shoulders farther from the floor. Your back will now lift off of the floor. Keep your knees bent. In the beginning, it may help to place your feet under a heavy chair or some other restraint. Once your abdominal muscles are strong enough, this should not be necessary and not done, because it allows your legs to help the abdomen in allowing you to raise. The motion should be a gentle smooth curling and uncurling. Never jerk to achieve greater height or an additional repetition and never strain or exert beyond reasonable comfort. Again, start with three repetitions and progress to at least ten.

25. Advanced Sit-up

Objective. Maximally strengthen low back and abdominal muscles.

Basic Exercise. Lie on your back on a covered floor with your knees well bent. Squeeze your buttocks and tighten your abdominal muscles. Start with your arms folded over your waist and smoothly lift your head, shoulders and back up to a position where your arms are touching your knees. Hold ten seconds, return to the starting position, relax a few seconds and then repeat. Again, start with three repetitions and progress to at least ten.

26. Advanced Modified Sit-up

Objective. Maximally strengthen low back and abdominal muscles.

Basic Exercise. Progress gradually until ten of the basic-advanced sit-ups can be easily and comfortably executed. Then try folding the arms in front of your face instead of your waist. As you curl up to your knees, hold ten seconds, then return to the starting position, relax a few seconds and repeat. Start with three repetitions. When this modified version can be accomplished ten times, you are ready to attempt a sit-up with your hands clasped behind your head. When this version can also be done ten times, you may, if desired, attempt the most difficult version of a sit-up. This involves lying on your back on a padded, inclined surface (i.e., a tilt board with the foot end elevated). Knees bent, hands clasped behind your neck, slowly and carefully execute the sit-up, hold ten seconds, slowly uncurl to the starting position, relax and repeat. The more inclined the board, the greater strength and effort will be required of your back and abdomen to accomplish the sit-up.

27. Sitting Bend

Objective. Strengthen your low back while stretching your low back and hamstring muscles.

Basic Exercise. Sit on a hard chair, feet flat on the floor, knees not more than 12 inches apart, arms folded loosely in your lap. Squeeze buttocks and tighten abdominal muscles so that your back goes flat against the chair. Bend over letting your head go between your knees with your elbows pointing toward the floor. Bend as far as is comfortable, hold for a count of five, then slowly pull your body back to the flat back sitting starting position. Relax a few seconds, repeat three times, gradually increasing to ten repetitions.

28. Divers Stance

Objective. Improve balance and posture while strengthening extensor muscles of the legs and feet.

Basic Exercise. Stand erect with your buttocks and abdomen tensed, feet slightly apart, and your arms at your sides. Lift up on your toes while raising your arms upward and forward, so they are extended palms down at shoulder height, parallel to the floor. Hold this position for ten seconds then return to the starting position and repeat.

29. Deep Knee Bend

Objective. Strengthen hamstring and quadraceps muscles.
   CAUTION: Do not begin this exercise until you can do a good back flattener. Have someone confirm that you are indeed holding your back flat while executing exercise No. 6. Most should not attempt this exercise until a month into this exercise program. Discontinue the exercise if there is considerable, lasting discomfort in your knees or hips.)

Basic Exercise. Stand behind a sofa, desk, heavy chair, or similar structure holding onto it for balance. Squeeze and tighten your buttocks and abdomen. Slowly bend your knees and, with a flat back, squat down as far as is reasonably comfortable; then stand up using only your legs, not your arms. Relax for a second or two and then do three repetitions, gradually building up to ten repetitions.

Table A–4

Strenuous Activities (7–10 K Cal/min, 150-lb person)

1. Chopping wood
2. Digging holes
3. Shoveling snow
4. Shoveling dirt, sand, manure, etc.
5. Walking up steep hills
6. Carrying anything weighing over 50 lb
7. Carrying anything weighing between 30–50 lb up an incline
8. Walking up stairs
9. Walking up hills
10. Any activity from Table A–5 done at a very vigorous pace so as to produce deep breathing and a concomitant rise in heart rate to 120–130 per minute.

Table A–5
Moderately Strenuous Activities (4–6 K Cal/min,
150-lb person)

1. Mowing the lawn with a hand mower
2. Hoeing
3. Spading the garden
4. Raking leaves
5. Pulling weeds
6. Energetic playing of musical instrument
7. Sawing wood by hand
8. Splitting logs by hand
9. Vigorously mopping or scrubbing the floor
10. Walking up small hills
11. Walking in water
12. Walking in loose sand on the level
13 Pushing a loaded wheelbarrow
14. Carrying anything weighing between 30–50 lb on the level
15. Painting requiring constant movement and going up and down
    a ladder
16. Cutting the hedges with non-electric clippers
17. Sanding wood, metal, etc.
18. Any activity from Table A–6 done at a very vigorous pace

Table A–6
Minimally Strenuous Activities (1–3 K Cal/min, 150-lb person)

1. Making the bed
2. Cleaning the tub
3. Ironing clothes
4. Putting groceries away
5. Vacuuming the floor or swimming pool
6. Dusting
7. Washing clothes by hand
8. Washing floors, walls, or windows
9. Light gardening
10. Mowing the lawn with a power mower
11. Pruning bushes
12. Cutting hedges with electric cutter
13. Washing the car
14. Waxing the car by hand
15. Making minor repairs on the car
16. Building with wood
17. Painting
18. Shampooing rugs with electric cleaner
19. Any activity requiring walking on a level or downhill surface
20. Raking leaves
21. Paper hanging
22. Brick laying
23. Cleaning windows
24. Light carpentry
25. Janitorial work
26. Sewing, knitting
27. Playing a musical instrument

Table A-7
Recreational Sports

	Light	Light-moderate	Moderate	Heavy
Archery*		X	X	
Badminton*		X	X	
Basketball			X	
Bicycling*		X (on level; easy pace)	X	X (briskly or uphill)
Billiards*	X	X		
Boccie*+		X		
Bowling*+		X	X	
Canoeing*		X	X	
Croquet*		X		
Cross-country skiing			X	X
Curling*			X	
Dancing*		X	X	
Darts*		X		
Deck tennis*			X	
Fencing			X	
Fishing*	X	X	X	X (deep-sea fishing)
Golf*		X (with cart)	X (without cart)	
Handball			X	X
Horseback riding*		X	X	
Horseshoes*+		X		
Jogging			X	X
Mountain climbing			X	X
Paddle tennis			X	
Putting*		X		
Quoits+	X			
Rowing*		X	X	
Sailing*		X		
Shooting*		X		
Shuffleboard*	X	X		
Skating*			X	
Skindiving		X	X	
Softball			X	

203

Table A-7 Continued

	Light	Light-moderate	Moderate	Heavy
Squash			X	X
Swimming*			X (breast stroke)	X (overhand crawl)
Table tennis*			X	
Tennis*			X (doubles)	X (singles)
Touch football			X	
Volleyball*		X	X	
Walking*		X (on level; slow pace)	X (on level; briskly)	X (up stairs or uphill)
Waterskiing			X	X

*Recommended for person over 50 by the International Committee on the Standardization of Physical Fitness.
+Should be approached cautiously by those with back problems.

204

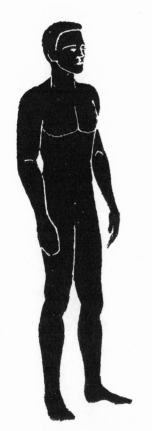
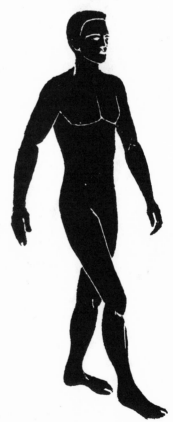

Walk.

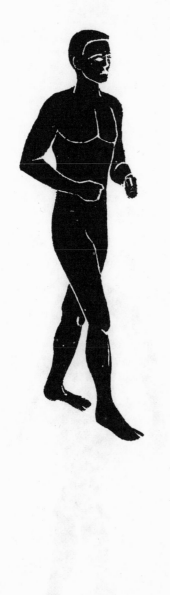
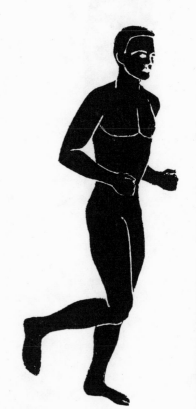

Alternate Walk-Jog.

Figure A–3

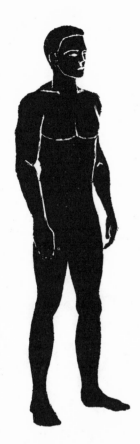

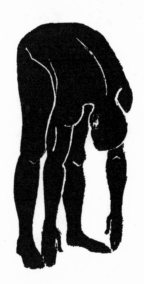

Bend and Stretch.

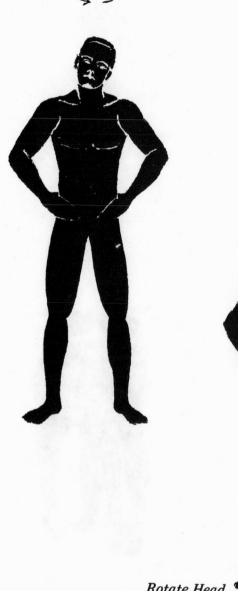

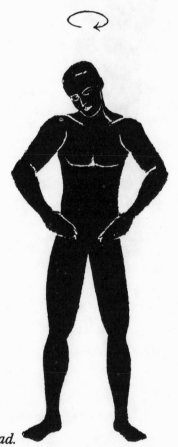

Rotate Head.

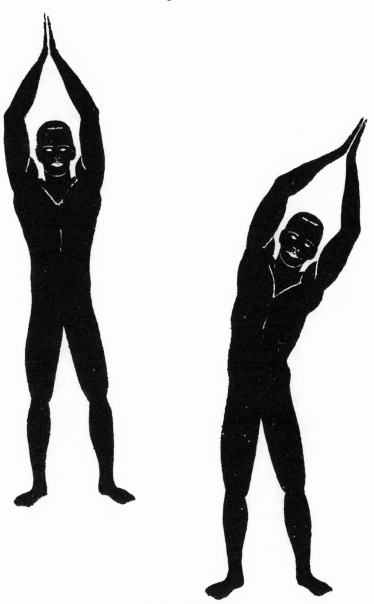

Body Bender.

209

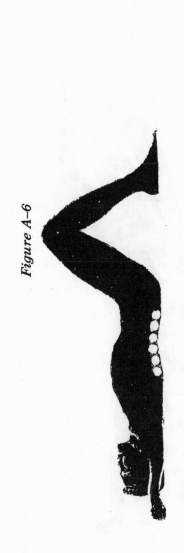

Figure A–6

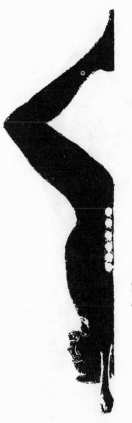

Back Flattener.

Figure A-7

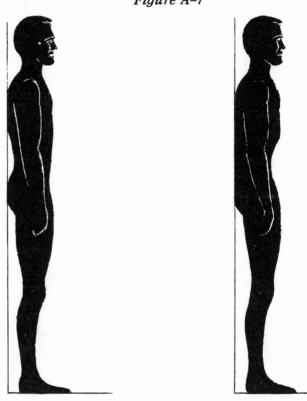

Wall Press.

Figure A–8

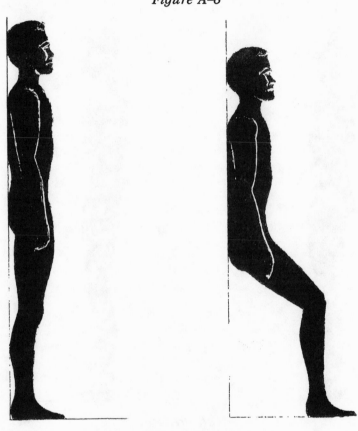

Posture Check.

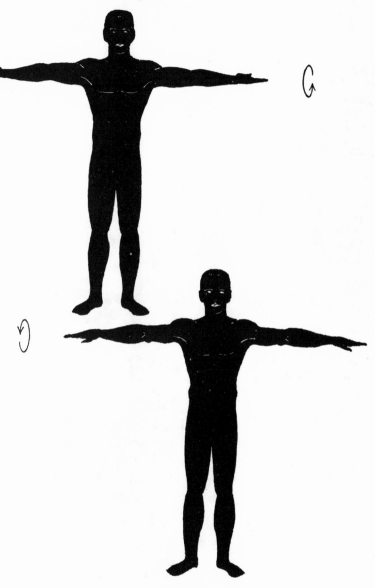

Arm Circles.

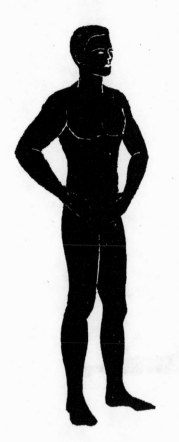

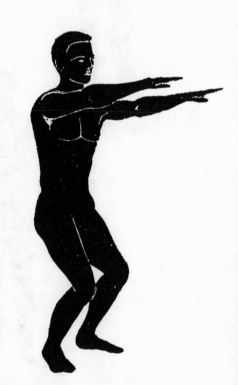

Half Knee Bend.

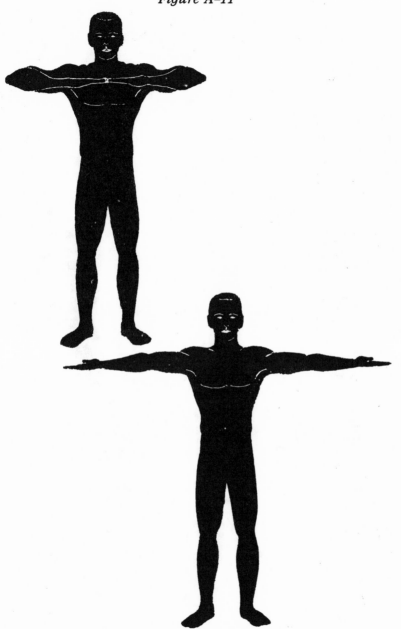

Wing Stretcher.

Figure A–12

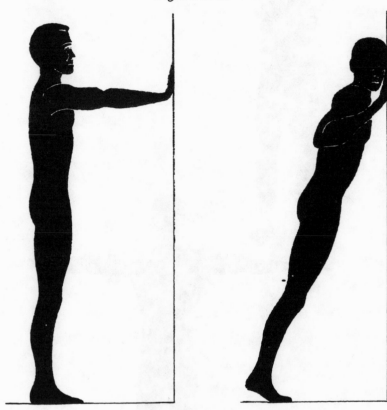

Wall Push-up.

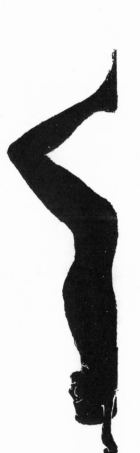

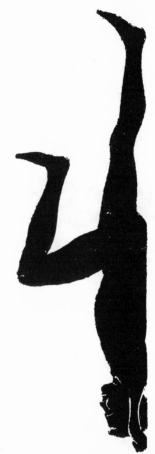

Single Knee Raise.

217

Figure A–14

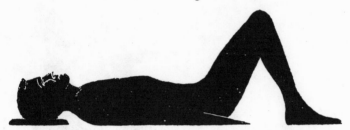

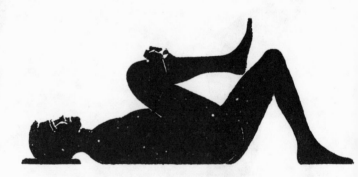

Single Knee Hug.

Figure A–15

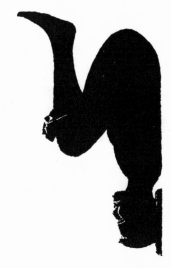

Double Knee Hug.

Figure A-16

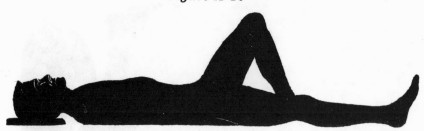

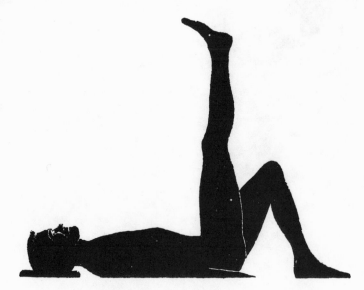

Single Leg Raise.

Figure A–17

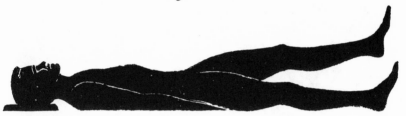

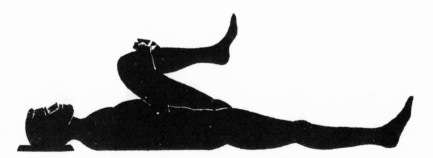

Single Leg Raise and Knee Hug.

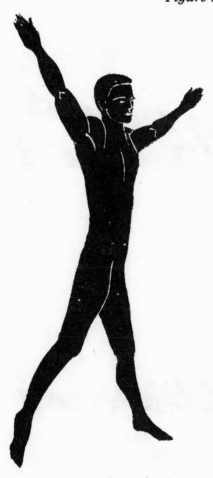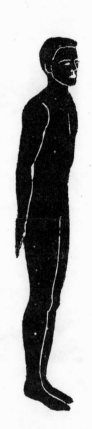

Straight Arm and Leg Stretch.

Figure A–19

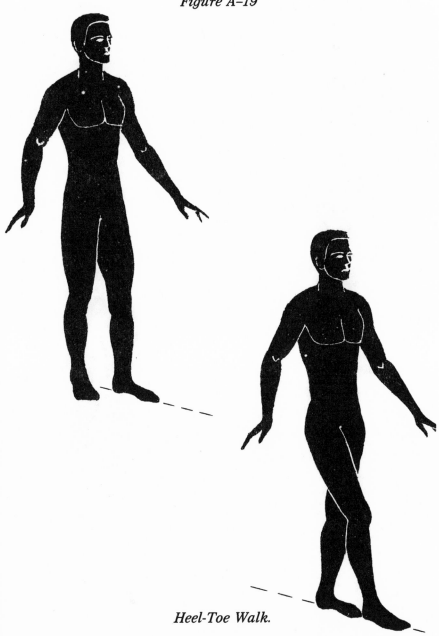

Heel-Toe Walk.

223

Figure A-20

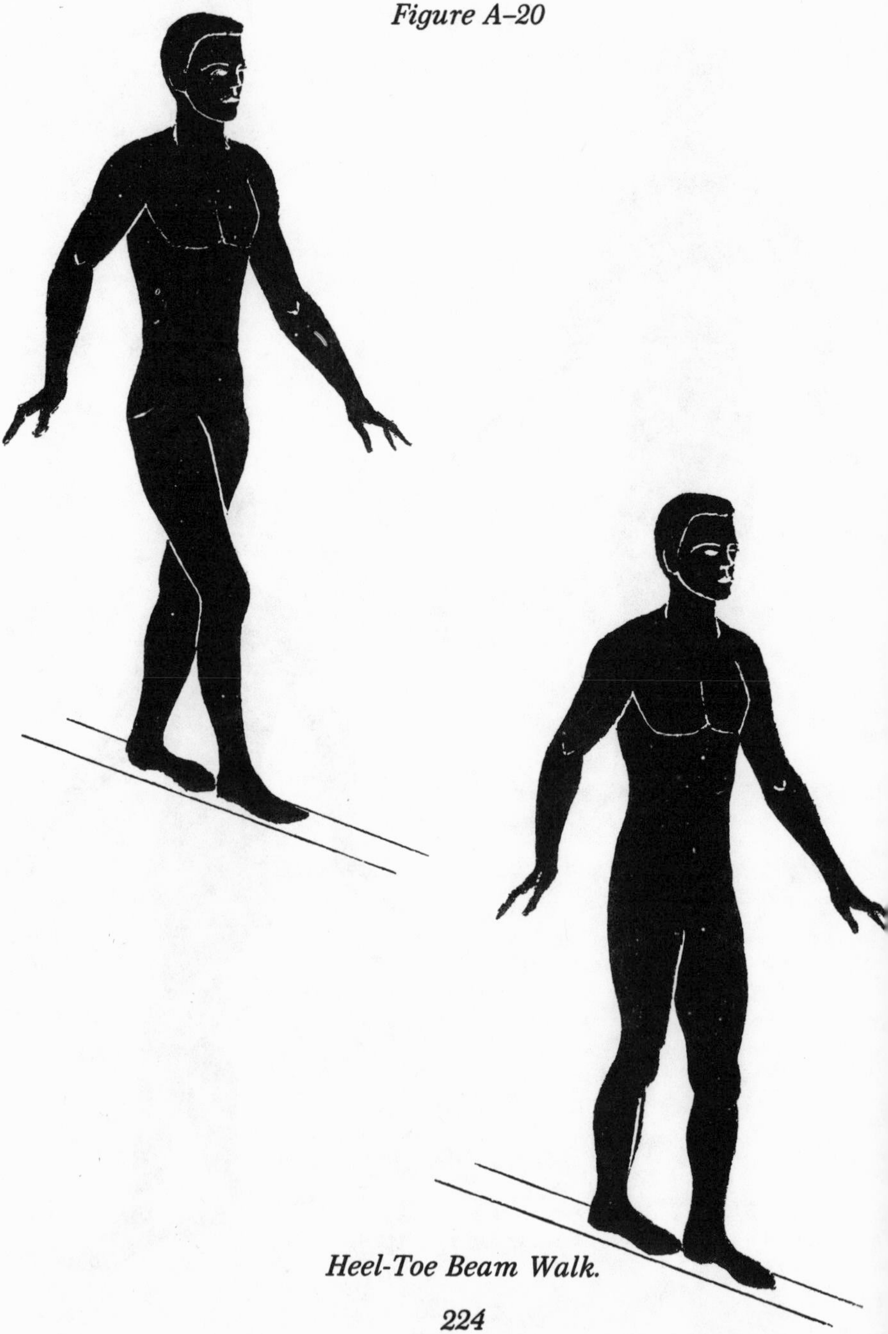

Heel-Toe Beam Walk.

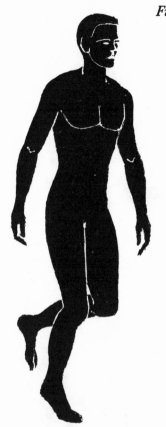

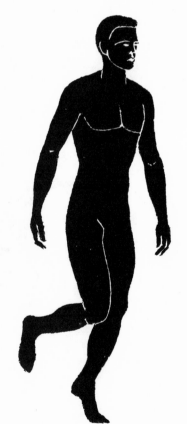

Hop.

Figure A–22

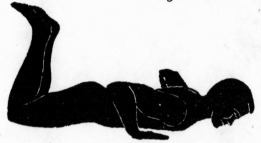

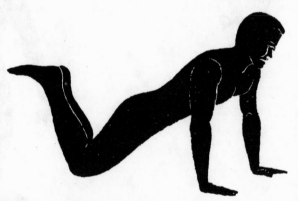

Knee Push-up.

Figure A-23

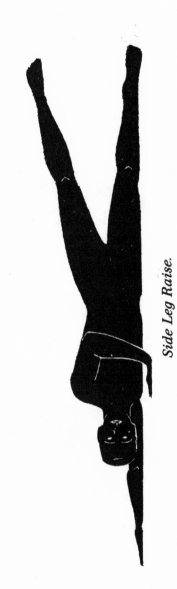

Side Leg Raise.

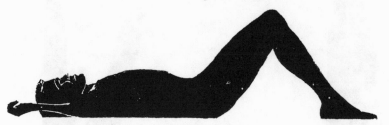

Figure A–24

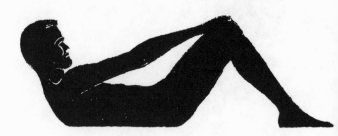

Partial Sit-up.

Figure A–25

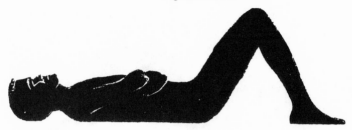

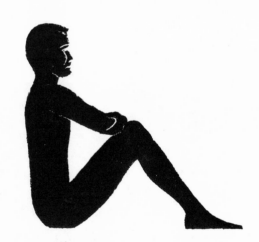

Advanced Sit-up.

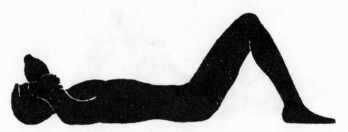

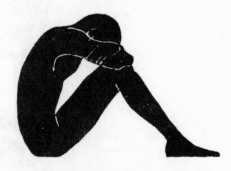

Advanced Modified Sit-up.

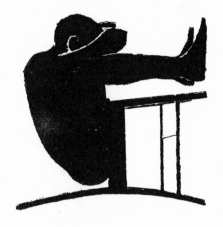

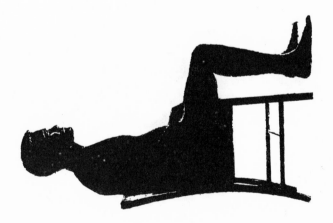

Sitting Bend.

Figure A–28

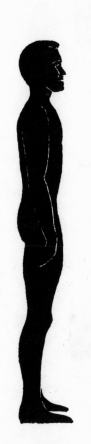

Divers Stance.

Figure A–29

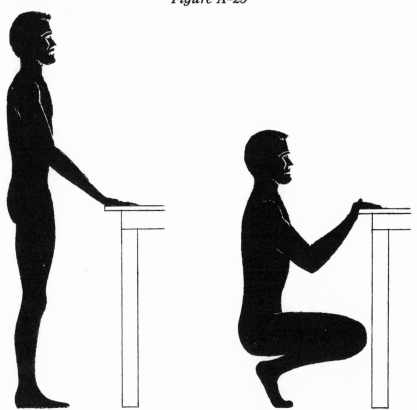

Deep Knee Bend.

References

CHAPTER 1

1. Anderson B., and Henderson J., (eds.): *Guide to Distance Running,* California, World Publications, 1971.
2. Barndt, R. Jr., Blankenhorn, D. H., Crawford, D. W., and Brooks, S. H.: "Regression and progression of early femoral atherosclerosis in treated hyperlipoproteinemic patients." *Annuals of Internal Medicine,* 86:139–146, 1977.
3. Bassler, T. J.: "Marathon running and immunity to heart disease." *Physician and Sports Medicine,* 3:77–80, 1975.
4. Cooper, K. H.: *Aerobics:* New York, M. Evans & Co., Inc., 1968.
5. Cooper, K. H.: *The New Aerobics:* New York, Bantam, 1970.
6. Cooper, K. H.: *The Aerobics Way* New York, M. Evans & Co., Inc., 1977.
7. Friedman, M., and Rosenman, R. H.: *Type A Behavior and Your Heart,* New York, Alfred A. Knopf, 1974.
8. Higdon, H.: *Fitness After Forty,* California, World Publications, 1977.
9. Kannel, W. B., Brand, N., Skinner, S. S., et. al.: "The relationship of adiposity to blood pressure and development of

hypertension: The Framingham Study." *Annuals of Internal Medicine,* 67:48–59, 1967.

10. Kannel, W. B., Dawber, T. R., Friedman, G. D., Glennon, W. E. and MacNamara, P. M.: "Risk factors in coronary heart disease: An evaluation of several serum lipids as predictors of coronary heart disease: The Framingham Study." *Annuals of Internal Medicine,* 61:888–899, 1964.

11. Kannel, W. B., Gordon, T., Sorlie, P., and MacNamara, P. M.: "Physical activity and coronary vulnerability; The Framingham Study." *Cardiology Digest,* 6:24–40, 1971.

12. Kannel, W. B. and Gordon, T. (eds.): *The Framingham Study: An Epidemiological Investigation of Cardiovascular Disease.* Section 30: Some characteristics related to the incidence of cardiovascular disease and death. Framingham Study, 19 year followup. Washington: Department of Health, Education and Welfare (National Institute of Health) 74–599, Feb. 1974.

13. Kannel, W. B. and Gordon, T. (eds.): *The Framingham Study: An Epidemiological Investigation of Cardiovascular Disease,* Washington, DHEW (NIH), 1968–1978, Sections 1–3.

14. Kavanaugh, T.: *Heart Attack? Counterattack!,* Toronto, Van Nostrand Reinhold Ltd, 1976.

15. Kostrubala, T.: *The Joy of Running,* New York, J. B. Lippincott Co., 1976.

16. Morris, J. W., Heady, J. A., Raffle, P. A., et. al.: "Coronary heart disease and physical activity of work." *Lancet,* 11:1053, 1953.

17. Morris, J. N., Chave, S. P., Adam, C., et. al.: "Vigorous exercise in leisure time and the incidence of coronary heart disease." *Lancet,* 1:333–339, 1973.

18. Paffenbarger, R. S., Jr.: "Hard work makes the heart grow safer." *New York Times,* March 24, p. 20, 1977.

19. Paffenbarger, R. S., Jr.: "Strenous exercise good heart medicine." *Enquirer and News,* Battle Creek, Mich., p. 85, November 28, 1977.

20. Spino, M.: *Beyond Jogging,* Millbrae, California. Celestial Arts, 1976.

CHAPTER 2

1. Beyer, P. L., Flynn, M. A.: "Effects of high- and low-fiber diets on human feces." *Journal of the American Dietetic Association,* 72:271–276, 1978.

2. Bottiger, L. E., Carlson, L. A., Hultman, E., et al.: "Serum lipids in alcoholics." *Acta Medica Scandinavica,* 199:357–361, 1976.

3. Brown, M. S., Goldstein, J. L.: "Familial hypercholesterolemia: a genetic defect in the low-density lipoprotein receptor." *New England Journal of Medicine* 294:1386–1390, 1976.

4. Care, T. E., Koschinsky, T., Hayes, S. B., et al.: "A mechanism by which high density lipoproteins may slow the atherogenic process." *Lancet* 1:1315–1317, 1976.

5. Chiang, B. N., Perlman, L. V., Epstein, F. H.: "Overweight and hypertension: a review" *Circulation,* 39:403–421, 1969.

6. DeWeese, V. A.: "No such thing as 'localized' arteriosclerosis, say surgeons." *Journal American Medical Association,* 238:571, 1977.

7. Dyer, A., Stamler, J., Paul, O., et al.: "Alcohol, cardiovascular risk factors for coronary heart disease." *Circulation,* 48:950–958, 1973.

8. Fletch, A. P.: "The effect of weight reduction upon the blood pressure of obese hypertensive." *Quarterly Journal of Medicine,* 23:331–345, 1954.

9. Heller, H. P., Hackler, L. R.: "Changes in the crude fiber content of the American diet." *American Journal of Clinical Nutrition,* 31:1510–1514, 1978.

10. Herbert, V.: Folic Acid and Vitamin B_{12}. Goodhart, R. S., Shile, M. E. (eds.): *Modern Nutrition in Health and Disease,* Philadelphia, Lea, & Febiger, 1973.

11. Hirst, A. E., Hadley, G. G., Gore, I.: "The effect of chronic alcoholism and cirrhosis of the liver on atherosclerosis." *American Journal of Medical Science,* 249:143–149, 1969.

12. Hrubec, Z.: "Coffee drinking and ischemic heart disease." *Lancet,* 1:548, 1973.

13. Jick, H., Miettinen, O. S., Neff, R. K., et al.: "Coffee and myocardial infarction." *New England Journal of Medicine,* 289:63–67, 1973.

14. Kannel, W. B., Brand, N., Skinner, J. J. et al.: "The relationship of adiposity to blood pressure and development of hypertension: The Framingham Study." *Annuals of Internal Medicine,* 67:48–59, 1967.

15. Kannel, W. B.: "Coffee, cocktails and coronary candidates." *New England Journal of Medicine,* 297:443–444, 1977.

16. Kavanaugh, T.: *Heart Attack? Counter Attack!,* Toronto, Van Nostrand Reinhold Ltd., 1976.

17. Lieber, C. S.: "Pathogenesis and early diagnosis of alcoholic liver injury." *New England Journal of Medicine,* 298:888–893, 1978.

18. Mann, G. V.: "The influence of obesity on health." *New England Journal of Medicine,* 291:178–185, 226–232, 1974.

19. *Massachusetts General Hospital Laboratory Newsletter,* Vol. II No. 1, 1977.

20. Montoye, H. G., Block, W., Keller, J. B., and Willis, P. W.: "Fitness, fatness, and serum cholesterol: an epidemiological study of an entire community." *The Research Quarterly,* 47:400–407, 1976.

21. Munoz, J. M., et al.: "Effects of some cereal brans and textured vegetable protein on plasma lipids." *American Journal of Clinical Nutrition,* 32:580–592, 1979.

22. Reisin, E., Abel, R., Molan, M., Silverberg, D. S., Eliahou, H. E., and Modan, B.: "Effect of weight loss without salt restriction on the reduction of blood pressure in overweight hypertensive patients." *New England Journal of Medicine,* 298:1–6, 1978.

23. Ross, R., Slomset, J. A.: "The pathogenesis of atherosclerosis." *New England Journal of Medicine,* 295:369–377, 420–425, 1976.

24. Small, D. M.: "Cellular mechanisms for lipid deposition in atherosclerosis." *New England Journal of Medicine,* 297:873–877, 1978.

25. Small, D. M.: "Cellular mechanisms for lipid deposition in

atherosclerosis." *New England Journal of Medicine,* 297:924–929, 1978.

26. Smith, D. A., Hawrysh, Z. J.: "Quality characteristics of wheat-bran chiffon cakes." *Journal of the American Dietetic Association,* 72:599–603, 1978.

27. Tobian, L.: "Hypertension and Obesity." *New England Journal of Medicine,* 298:46–48, 1978.

28. Tyroler, H. A., Heyden, S., Hames, C. G.: *Weight and hypertension: Evans County Study of Blacks and Whites, Epidemiology and Control of Hypertension.* Paul, O. (ed.), New York, Stratton Intercontinental, 1975.

29. Van Itallie, T. B., and Yang, M. U.: "Current concepts in nutrition diets and weight loss." *New England Journal of Medicine,* 297:1158–1161, 1977.

30. White, P. L.: "Vitamin preparations proper use in medical practice." *Postgraduate Medicine,* 60:204–209, 1976.

31. Yano, K., Rhoads, G. G., and Kagan, A.: "Coffee, Alcohol and risk of coronary heart disease among Japanese men living in Hawaii." *New England Journal of Medicine,* 297:405–409, 1977.

CHAPTER 3

1. Bray, G.: "Types of human obesity—a system of classification." *Obesity and Bariatric Medicine,* 2:147, 1973.

2. Bray, G. A. et al.: "Eating patterns of massively obese individuals." *Journal of the American Dietetic Association,* 72:24–30, 1978.

3. Chiang, B. N., Pearlman, L. V., Epstein, F. H.: "Overweight and hypertension: a review." *Circulation,* 39:403–421, 1969.

4. Franklin, B. A., Lussier, L., Buskirk, E. R.: "Injury rates in women joggers." *The Physician and Sports Medicine,* 17:105–112, 1979.

5. Goodman, C. E., Kenrick, M. M.: "Physical fitness in relation to obesity." *Obesity and Bariatric Medicine,* 4:12–12, 1975.

6. Kannel, W. B., Bond, N., Skinner, J. J., et al.: "The relationship of adiposity to the blood pressure and development of

hypertension. The Framingham Study." *Annuals of Intern. Med.,* 67:48–59, 1962.

7. Lieber, C. S.: "Pathogenesis and early diagnosis of alcoholic liver injury." *New England Journal of Medicine,* 298:888–893, 1978.

8. Mayer, J.: *Overweight,* Englewood Cliffs, Prentice-Hall 1968, pp. 100–115.

9. Pollock, M. L., Gettman, L. R., Milesis, C. A., et al.: "Effects of frequency and duration of training on attrition and incidence of injury." *Medicine in Science and Sports,* 91:31–36, 1977.

10. Schneider, H. A., Anderson, C. E., Coursin, D. B.: *Nutritional Support of Medical Practice,* Hagerstown, Maryland, Harper & Row, Publishers Inc., 1977.

11. Seltzer, C., Stare, F.: "Obesity: how it is measured, what causes it, how to treat it." *Medical Insight,* 10, 1973.

12. Stewart, R.: "Exercise prescriptions in weight management: advantages, techniques, and obstacles." *Obesity and Bariatric Medicine,* 4:21, 1975.

13. Stunkard, A., McLaren-Hume, M.: "The results of treatment for obesity. A review of the literature and report of a series." *Archives Internal Medicine,* 03:84, 1959.

14. Tobian, L.: "Hypertension and obesity." *New England Journal of Medicine,* 298:46–48, 1978.

15. Tyroler, H. A., Heyden, S., Homes, C. G.: Weight and hypertension. *Evans County Study of Whites and Blacks, Epidemiology and Control of Hypertension.* Paul, O. (ed.), New York, Stratton Intercontinental, 1975.

16. Tullis, F., Tullis, K. F.: Obesity. *Nutritional Support of Medical Practice.* Maryland, Harper and Row, 1977, pp. 392–406.

17. Walker, A. R. P.: "The relative risks of saccharin and sucrose solutions." *American Journal of Clinical Nutrition,* 32:727–728, 1979.

18. *Weight, Height, and Selected Body Dimensions of Adults,* Washington, D.C., U. S. Public Health Service, Government Printing Office, document #13247, 1965.

19. White, P.: "The dangers in diet advice." *Medical Insight,* July–August :30, 1973.

CHAPTER 4

1. Ahlborg, G., Felig, P., Hagenfeldt, L., Hendler, R., and Wahren, J.: "Substrate turnover during prolonged exercise in man." *Journal of Clinical Investigation,* 53:1080, 1974.

2. Angelov, I.: "Study of the interrelationship of glycemia—nonestinfied fatty acids in physical activity in diabetics." *Vutreshni Bolesti,* 15:76-80, 1976.

3. Berger, M.: "Muscular work in the therapy of diabetes mellitus." *Fortschritte der Medizin,* 94:1553–7, 1976.

4. Bierman, E. L., Albrink, M. J., Arky, R. A., et al.: "Special report: Principles of nutrition and dietary recommendations for patients with diabetes mellitus." *Diabetes,* 20:633–634, 1971.

5. Biermann, J., and Toohey, B.: *The Diabetic's Sports & Exercise Book,* New York, J. B. Lippincott Co., 1977.

6. Bircak, J., Michalkova, D., Silesova, J., Hudakova, G., Moravcikova, B., Rutt Kayova, R.: "Muscular and Metabolic changes in child diabetes." *Pediatrics,* 32:213–215, 1977.

7. Bjortorp, P., Fahlen, M., Grimby, G., et al.: "Carbohydrate and lipid metabolism in middle-aged, physically trained men." *Metabolism,* 21:1037–1044, 1972.

8. Craighead, J. E.: "Workshop on viral infection and diabetes mellitus in man." *Journal of Infectious Diseases,* 125:568–570, 1972.

9. Craighead, J. E.: "The role of viruses in the pathogenesis of pancreatic disease and diabetes mellitus." *Progress in Medical Virology,* 19:161–214, 1975.

10. Dorchy, H., et al.: "Effect of exercise on glucose uptake in diabetic adolescents." *Acta Paediatrica Belgica,* 29:83–85, 1976.

11. Felig, P. and Wahen, J.: "Fuel homeostasis in exercise." *New England Journal of Medicine,* 293:1078–84, 1975.

12. Florey, C. D., McDonald, H., Miall, W. E., et al.: "Serum lipids and their relation to blood glucose and cardiovascular measurements in a rural population of Jamaican adults." *Chronic Diseases,* 26:85–100, 1973.

13. Gabbay, K.: "New Directions in Diabetes." *Childrens World,* 4:2–17, 1977.

14. Gamble, D. R., Taylor, K. W., Cummings, H.: "Coxsackie viruses and diabetes mellitus." *British Medical Journal,* 4:260–262, 1973.

15. Guthrie, D. W.: "Exercise, diets and insulin for child with diabetes." *Nursing,* 7:48–54, 1977.

16. Hawkins, B.: "Running sweetens the diabetic's life." *Runners World,* May, 1977.

17. Hempfer, P.: "Sport and movement the most important vital help for the diabetic children." *Schweizerische Zeitschrift fur Sportmedizin,* 22:141–149, 1974.

18. Izumi, K., Itoh, K. F., and Shigeta, Y.: Dietary Treatment of Japanese Diabetics: Management of Hyperlipemia. *Diabetes Mellitus in Asia.* Baba, S., et al., Amsterdam, Exerpta Medica, 1976.

19. Kawamore, R., Vranic, M.: "Mechanism of exercise-induced hypoglycemia in depancreatized dogs maintained on long-acting insulin." *Journal of Clinical Investigation,* 59:331–337, 1977.

20. Kawate, R., Miyaniski, M., and Nishimoto, Y.: Prevalence and Mortality of Diabetes Mellitus in Japanese in Hawaii and Japan. *Diabetes Mellitus in Asia.* Baba, S., et al. Amsterdam, Exerpta Medica, 1976.

21. Koivisto, V. A., and Felig, P.: "Effects of leg exercise on insulin absorption in diabetic patients." *New England Journal of Medicine,* 298:79–83, 1978.

22. Kuzuya, T., Irie, M., and Nila, Y.: Glucose Intolerance Among Japanese Professional Sumo-wrestlers. *Diabetes Mellitus in Asia.* Baba, S., et al. Amsterdam, Exerpta Medica, 1976.

23. Maehlum, S.: "Muscular exercise and metabolism in male juvenile diabetics. II Glucose tolerance after exercise."

Scandanavian Journal of Clinical Laboratory Investigation, 32:145–153, 1973.

24. Maehlum, S., Jervell & Ester, S., and Pruett, D. R.: "Arterial-hepatic vein glucose differences in normal and diabetic man after a glucose infusion at rest and after exercise." *Scandanavian Journal of Clinical Laboratory Investigation,* 36:415–22, 1976.

25. Mogensen, C. E., and Vittinghus, E.: "Urinary albumen excretion during exercise in juvenile diabetes." *Scandanavian Journal of Clinical Laboratory Investigation,* 35:295–300, 1975.

26. Murray, F. T., et al.: "The metabolic response to moderate exercise in diabetic man receiving intravenous and subcutaneous insulin." *Journal of Clinical Endocrinology and Metabolism,* 44:708–720, 1977.

27. Neel, J. V.: "The genetics of juvenile-onset-type diabetes mellitus." *New England Journal of Medicine,* 297:1062–1064, 1977.

28. Norlander, S., Ostman, J., Cerasi, E., Luft, R., and Ekelund, L. G.: "Occurrence of diabetic type of plasma FFA and glycerol responses to physical exercise in prediabetic subjects." *Acta Medica Scandanavica,* 193:9–21, 1973.

29. Ponikowska, I.: "Effect of graded physical exercise on blood sugar level in healthy subjects and diabetics." *Polski Tygodnik Lekarski,* 27:1961–1963, 1972.

30. Pruett, E. D. R., and Maehlum, S.: "Muscular exercise and metabolism in male juvenile diabetics." *Scandanavian Journal of Clinical Laboratory Investigation,* 32:139–147, 1973.

31. Rowell, I. B., Mesoro, E. J., and Spenser, M. S.: "Splanchnic metabolism in exercising man." *Journal of Applied Physiology,* 20:1032, 1965.

32. Rubinstein, P., Suciu-Foca, W., and Nicholson, J. F.: "Genetics of juvenile diabetes mellitus." *New England Journal of Medicine,* 297:1036–1040, 1977.

33. Truswell, A. S., and Mann, J. I.: "Epidemiology of serum lipids in Southern Africa." *Atherosclerosis,* 16:15–29, 1972.

34. Vogelberg, K. H., et al.: "The treatment of chronic insulin

resistance in adipose diabetics-interruption for a short time of diet and administration." *Muenchener Medizinische Wochenschrift,* 118:1037–1040, 1976.

35. Wahren, J., Felig, P., Ahlborg, G., et al.: "Glucose metabolism during leg exercise in man." *Journal of Clinical Investigation,* 50:2715–2725, 1971.

36. Wahren, J., Hagenfeldt, L., Felig, P.: "Glucose and free fatty acid utilization in exercise studies in normal and diabetic man." *Israel Journal of Medical Science,* 11:551–559, 1975.

37. Wahren, J., Hagenfeldt, L., and Felig, P.: "Splanchnic and leg exchange of glucose, amino acids, and free fatty acids during exercise in diabetes mellitus." *Journal of Clinical Investigation,* 55:1303, 1975.

38. West, K. M., and Kalbfleisch, J. M.: "Diabetes in Central America." *Diabetes,* 19:656–663, 1970.

39. West, K. M., and Kalbfleisch, J. M.: "Influence of nutritional factors on prevalence of diabetes." *Diabetes,* 20:99–108, 1971.

40. West, K. M.: "Epidemiologic evidence linking nutritional factors to the prevalence and manifestation of diabetes." *Diabetologia,* 9:405–428, 1972.

41. ———.: "Diet therapy of diabetes: An analysis of failure." *Annuals Internal Medicine,* 79:425–434, 1973.

42. ———.: "Diabetes in American Indians and other native populations of the new world." *Diabetes,* 23:841–855, 1974.

43. ———.: Epidemiologic Observations on Thirteen Populations of Asia and the Western Hemisphere. *Proceedings of VIII International Sugar Research Foundation,* S. S. Hillebrand, (ed.), 1974, pp. 33–43.

44. ———.: "Prevention and therapy of diabetes mellitus." *Nutritional Review,* 33:193–198, 1975.

45. ———.: "Diet and diabetes." *Postgraduate medicine,* 60:209–16, 1976.

46. White, P. L.: "Diet and Health—Vitamine Preparations." *Postgraduate Medicine,* 60:204–209, 1976.

CHAPTER 5

1. Akeson, W. H., and Murphy, R. W. (ed.): "Clinical orthopedics and related research." *Comment,* 129:2–3, 1977.

2. Ferguson, R. J.: "Low back pain in college football linemen." *Journal of Sports Medicine,* 2:63–80, 1974.

3. Friedmann, L. W., and Galton, L.: *Freedom From Backaches,* New York, Pocket Books, 1973.

4. Distenfano, A.: "Injuries to the low back and environs." *Athletic Training* 11, page 169.

5. Harris, W. D.: "Low back pain in sports medicine." *Journal of the Arkansas Medical Society,* 74:377–379, 1978.

6. Jones, L.: *The Postural Complex,* Springfield, Ill., C. C. Thomas, 1955.

7. Kahn, E. A., Crosby, E. C., Schneider, R. C., and Taren, J. A.: *Correlative Neurosurgery,* Springfield, Ill., Charles C. Thomas, 1969.

8. Kraus, H.: *Backache Stress And Tension,* New York, Simon and Schuster, 1965.

9. Meyerding, H. W.: "Low backache and sciatic pain associated with spondylolisthesis and protruded intervertebral disc: incidence, significance, and treatment." *Journal of Bone and Joint Surgery,* 23:461–470, 1941.

10. Root, L., and Kiernan, T.: *Oh, My Aching Back,* New York, New American Library, 1975.

11. Ruge, D., and Wiltse, L. L.: *Spinal Disorders,* Philadelphia, Lea and Febiger, 1977.

12. Smith, C. F.: "Physical management of muscular low back pain in the athlete." *Canadian Medical Journal,* 177:632–635, 1977.

CHAPTER 7

1. Abramson, J. H. and Hopp, C.: "The control of cardiovascular risk factors in the elderly." *Preventive Medicine,* 5:32–37, 1976.

2. Amsterdam, E. A., Wilmore, J. H., and DeMaria, A. N.: *Exercise in Cardiovascular Health and Disease,* New York, Yorke Medical Books, 1977.

3. Corday, E. and Corday, S. R.: "Prevention of heart disease by control of risk factors; the time has come to face the facts." *American Journal of Cardiology,* 35:330–333, 1975.

4. Dawber, T. R., and Kannel, W. B.: "Current status of coronary prevention, lesson learned from the Framingham Study." *Preventive Medicine,* 1:499–512, 1972.

5. Elmfeldt, D., Wilhelmsen, L., Wedel, H., Vedin, A., Wilhelmsson, C., and Tibblin, G.: "Primary risk factors in patients with myocardial infarction." *New England Journal of Medicine,* 91:412–419, 1976.

6. Fox, S. M., Naughton, J. P., and Gorman, P. A.: "Physical activity and cardiovascular health. The exercise prescription; frequency and type of activity." *Modern Concepts of Cardiovascular Disease,* 41:25, 1972.

7. Glancy, D. L.: "Exercise stress testing in patients suspected of having ischemic heart disease." *Journal of Louisiana State Medical Society,* 129:27–34, 1977.

8. Hirsch, E. Z., Hellerstein, H. K., and Macleod, C. A.: Physical Straining and Coronary Heart Disease. *Exercise and the Heart Guidelines for Exercise Programs,* Morse, R. L., ed., Springfield, Ill., Thomas, 1972, Chapt. 8, p. 106.

9. Kagan, R.: "Atherosclerosis and myocardial disease in relation to physical activity of occupation." *Bulletin World Health Organization,* 53:615–672, 1976.

10. Kannel, W. B., Dawber, T. R., Friedman, G. D., Glennon, W. E., and MacNamara, P. M.: "Risk factors in coronary heart disease: An evaluation of several serum lipids as predictors of coronary heart disease: The Framingham Study." *Annuals of Internal Medicine,* 61:888–899, 1964.

11. Kannel, W. B., Gordon, T., Sorlie, P., and MacNamara, P. M.: "Physical activity and coronary vulnerability: The Framingham Study." *Cardiology Digest,* 6:24–40, 1971.

12. Kannel, W. B. and Gordon, T. (eds.): *The Framingham Study: An Epidemiological Investigation of Cardiovascular*

Disease. Some Characteristics Related To the Incidence of Cardiovascular Disease and Death. Framingham Study 18 year follow-up. Washington, *Department of Health, Education and Welfare (National Institute of Health)* Feb. 1974, 74–599.

13. Kannel, W. B. and Gordon, T. (eds.): *The Framingham Study: An Epidemiological Investigation of Cardiovascular Disease.* Washington, *Department of Health, Education and Welfare (National Institute of Health)* 1968–1975, Sections 1–3.

14. Kasch, F. W., Phillips, W. H., Carter, J. E. L., et al.: "Cardiovascular changes in middle-aged men during two years of training." *Journal of Applied Physiology,* 34:53–57, 1973.

15. Kavanaugh, T.: *Heart Attack? Counter Attack!,* Toronto, Van Nostrand Reinhold Ltd., 1976.

16. Kiell, P. J.: *Keep Your Heart Running,* New York, Winchester Press, 1976.

17. Kirchleiner, B., and Pedersen-Bjergaard, O.: "The effect of physical training after myocardial infarction." *Scand. Society of Rehabilitative Medicine,* 5:105–110, 1973.

18. Mann, G. V., et al.: "Exercise to prevent coronary heart disease: an experimental study of the effects of training on risk factors for coronary heart disease in man." *American Journal of Medicine,* 46:12, 1969.

19. Margolis, S.: "Physician strategies for the prevention of coronary heart disease." *The Johns Hopkins Medical Journal,* 141:170–176, 1977.

20. Masters, A. M., and Rosenfeld, I.: "Exercise electrocardiography as an estimation of cardiac function." *Diseases of Chest,* 51:347, 1967.

21. Merriman, J. E.: Long-term Activity Programs For Coronary Patients. *Exercise Testing and Exercise Training in Coronary Heart Disease,* Naughton, J., and Hellerstein, H. K., (eds.), New York, Academic Press, 1973.

22. Michael, E., Evert, J., and Jeffers, K.: "Physiological changes of teenage girls during months of detraining." *Medicine and Science in Sports,* 4:241, 1972.

23. Morris, J. N., Heady, J. A., Raffle, P. A., et al.: "Coronary heart disease and physical activity of work." *Lancet,* 11:1053, 1953.

24. Naughton, J. P., and Hellerstein, H. K.: *Exercise Testing and Exercise Training in Coronary Heart Disease,* New York, Academic Press, 1973, pp. 253–262.

25. Siegel, W., Blomquist, G., and Mitchell, J. H.: "Effects of a quantitated physical training program on middle-aged sedentary males." *Circulation,* 41:19, 1970.

26. Stein, R. A.: "The effect of exercise training on heart rate during coitus in the post myocardial infarction patient." 55:738–740, 1977.

27. Walker, W. J.: Letter to ed. regarding Diet-heart era: premature obituary, *New England Journal of Medicine,* 298:106–107, 1978.

28. Wilmore, J. H.: Individualized exercise prescription. *Exercise Testing and Exercise Training in Coronary Heart Disease,* Naughton, J. and Hellerstein, H. K. (eds.), New York, Academic Press, 1973.

29. Zohman, L. R.: "Exercise stress test interpretation for cardiac diagnosis and functional evaluation." *Archives of Physical Medicine and Rehabilitation,* 58:235–240, 1977.

CHAPTER 8

1. Boileau, R. A., Massey, B. H., and Misner, J. E.: "Body composition changes in adult men during selected weight training and jogging programs." *Research Quarterly,* 44:158–174, 1973.

2. Cantwell, J. D., and Watt, E. W.: "Extreme cardiopulmonary fitness in old age." *Chest,* 65:1974, pp. 357–358.

3. Cooper, K. H.: *Aerobics,* New York, M. Evans & Co. Inc., 1968.

4. ———. *The New Aerobics,* New York, Bantam, 1970.

5. ———. *The Aerobics Way,* New York, M. Evans & Co. Inc., 1977.

6. Flint, M. M., Drinkwater, B. L., and Horvath, S. M.: "Effects

of training on women's response to submaximal exercise." *Medicine and Science in Sports,* 6:1974, 89–94.

7. Getchell, L. H., and Moore, J. C.: "Physical training comparative responses of middle-aged adults." *Archives of Physical Medical Rehabilitation,* 56:250–254, 1975.

8. Guber, S., Montoye, H. J., Cunningham, D. A., and Dinka, S. Jr.: "Age and physiological adjustment to continuous graded treadmill exercise." *Research Quarterly,* 43:175–184, 1972.

9. Horne, W. M.: "Effects of a physical activity program on middle-aged sedentary corporation executives." *Am. Indiana Hygiene Assoc. J.,* 36:241–245, 1975.

10. Jette, M., and Cureton, T. K.: "Anthropometric and selected motor fitness measurements of men engaged in a long-term program of physical activity." *Research Quarterly,* 47:667–671, 1976.

11. Kasch, F. W., and Boyer, J. L.: "Changes in maximum work capacity resulting from six month training in patients with ischemic heart disease." *Medicine and Science in Sports,* 1:156, 1969.

12. Kasch, F. W., Phillips, W. H., Carter, J. E. L., et al.: "Cardiovascular changes in middle-aged men during two years of training." *Journal of Applied Physiology,* 34:53–57, 1973.

13. Linnerud, A. C., and Ward, A.: "Follow-up study on the effects of conditioning four days per week on the physical fitness of adult men." *American Corrective Therapy Journal,* 28:135–139, 1974.

14. Liv, N., and Cureton, T. K. Jr.: "Effects of training on maximal oxygen intake of middle-aged women." *American Corrective Therapy Journal,* 29:56–61, 1975.

15. Mann, G. V., et al.: "Exercise to prevent coronary heart disease: an experimental study of the effects of training on risk factors for coronary heart disease in man." *American Journal of Medicine,* 46:12, 1969.

16. McDonough, J. R., Kusumi, F., and Bruce, R. A.: "Variations in maximal oxygen intake with physical activity in middle-aged men." *Circulation,* 41:743–751, 1970.

17. Park, R. J.: "Concern for health and exercise as expressed in

the writings of 18th century physicians and informed laymen (England, France, Switzerland)." *The Research Quarterly,* 47:756–766.

18. Pollock, M. L., Cureton, T. K., and Greninger, L.: "Effects of frequency of training on working capacity, cardiovascular function, and body composition of adult men." *Medicine in Science and Sports,* 1:70–74, 1969.

19. Pollock, M. L., Broida, J., Kendrick, Z., et al.: "Effect of training two days per week at different intensities of middle-aged men." *Medicine in Science and Sports,* 4:192–197, 1972.

20. Pollock, M. L.: The Quantification of Endurance Training Programs. *Exercise and Sport Sciences Reviews,* Wilmore, J. H. (ed.), New York, Academic Press, 1973, pp. 115–188.

21. Stoedefalke, K. G.: "Physical fitness programs for adults." *American Journal of Cardiology,* 33:787–790, 1974.

22. Van Handel, P. J., Costill, D. L., and Getchell, L. H.: "Central circulatory adaptations to physical training." *Research Quarterly of American Association Health and Physical Education,* 47:815–823, 1976.

23. Wilmore, J. H.: "Individual exercise prescription." *American Journal of Cardiology,* 33:757–759, 1974.

24. Wilmore, J. H., and Behnke, A. R.: "An anthropometric estimation of body density and lean body weight in young men." *Journal of Applied Physiology,* 27:25–31, 1969.

25. Young, J. R., and Ismail, A. H.: "Personality differences of adult men before and after a physical fitness program." *The Research Quarterly,* 47:513–519, 1976.

CHAPTER 9

1. Anderson, R. (ed.): *Runners World,* Cover page November, 1977.

2. Beverley, E. V.: "An assortment of fitness programs for the unconditioned retired." *Geriatrics,* 31:122–131, 1976.

3. Bolton, B., and Milligan, T.: "The effects of a systematic physical fitness program on clients in a comprehensive

rehabilitation center." *American Corrective Therapy Journal,* 30:41–46, 1976.

4. Currens, J. H., and White, P. D.: "Half a century of running: Clinical, physiologic and autopsy findings in the case of Clarence DeMar ("Mr. Marathon"). *New England Journal of Medicine,* 265:988–993, 1961.

5. deVries, H. A.: *Vigor regained. A Simple, Proven Home Program for Restoring Fitness and Vitality,* Engelwood Cliffs, New Jersey, Prentice-Hall Inc., 1974.

6. Lilliefors, J.: "John Kelley: a half century of racing." *Runners World,* November 1977, page 38.

7. Park, R. J.: "Concern for health and exercise as expressed in the writings of 18th century physicians and informed laymen (England, France, Switzerland)." *The Research Quarterly,* 47:756–767, 1976.

8. Proxmire, W.: *You Can Do It,* New York, Simon and Schuster, 1973.

9. Ranson, A. J.: "Swimming and cardiovascular fitness in the older age group." *Journal of Sports Medicine,* 3:35–40, 1975.

10. Shelly, E. L.: "A graded and monitored exercise program for senior adults." *Texas Medicine,* 72:58–63, 1976.

11. Suominen, H., Heikkinen, E., and Parkatti, T.: "Effect of eight weeks' physical training on muscle and connective tissue of the m. vastus lateralis in 69-year old men and women." *Journal of Gerontology,* 32:33–37, 1977.

12. Sussman, A., and Goode, R.: *The Magic of Walking,* New York, Simon and Schuster, Inc., 1967.

13. Winter, R.: *Ageless Aging: How to Extend Your Healthy and Productive Years,* New York, Crown Publishers Inc., 1973.

14. The Fitness Challenge in the Later Years. *Department of Health, Education and Welfare* Publication No. (Office of Health and Development) 75-20802, June, 1975.

Index